Toward Quality Measures
for Population Health
and the Leading
Health Indicators

Committee on Quality Measures for the Healthy People Leading
Health Indicators

Board on Population Health and Public Health Practice

INSTITUTE OF MEDICINE
OF THE NATIONAL ACADEMIES

THE NATIONAL ACADEMIES PRESS
Washington, D.C.
www.nap.edu

THE NATIONAL ACADEMIES PRESS • 500 Fifth Street, NW • Washington, DC 20001

NOTICE: The project that is the subject of this report was approved by the Governing Board of the National Research Council, whose members are drawn from the councils of the National Academy of Sciences, the National Academy of Engineering, and the Institute of Medicine.

This study was supported by Contract HHSP233201200032C between the National Academy of Sciences and the Department of Health and Human Services. Any opinions, findings, conclusions, or recommendations expressed in this publication are those of the authors and do not necessarily reflect the view of the organizations or agencies that provided support for this project.

International Standard Book Number-13: 978-0-309-28557-5
International Standard Book Number-10: 0-309-28557-7

Additional copies of this report are available from the National Academies Press, 500 Fifth Street, NW, Keck 360, Washington, DC 20001; (800) 624-6242 or (202) 334-3313; http://www.nap.edu.

For more information about the Institute of Medicine, visit the IOM home page at: **www.iom.edu.**

Suggested citation: IOM (Institute of Medicine). 2012. *Toward quality measures for population health and the leading health indicators.* Washington, DC: The National Academies Press.

"Knowing is not enough; we must apply.
Willing is not enough; we must do."

—Goethe

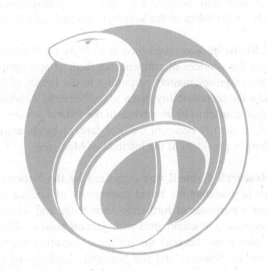

INSTITUTE OF MEDICINE
OF THE NATIONAL ACADEMIES

Advising the Nation. Improving Health.

THE NATIONAL ACADEMIES
Advisers to the Nation on Science, Engineering, and Medicine

The **National Academy of Sciences** is a private, nonprofit, self-perpetuating society of distinguished scholars engaged in scientific and engineering research, dedicated to the furtherance of science and technology and to their use for the general welfare. Upon the authority of the charter granted to it by the Congress in 1863, the Academy has a mandate that requires it to advise the federal government on scientific and technical matters. Dr. Ralph J. Cicerone is president of the National Academy of Sciences.

The **National Academy of Engineering** was established in 1964, under the charter of the National Academy of Sciences, as a parallel organization of outstanding engineers. It is autonomous in its administration and in the selection of its members, sharing with the National Academy of Sciences the responsibility for advising the federal government. The National Academy of Engineering also sponsors engineering programs aimed at meeting national needs, encourages education and research, and recognizes the superior achievements of engineers. Dr. C. D. Mote, Jr., is president of the National Academy of Engineering.

The **Institute of Medicine** was established in 1970 by the National Academy of Sciences to secure the services of eminent members of appropriate professions in the examination of policy matters pertaining to the health of the public. The Institute acts under the responsibility given to the National Academy of Sciences by its congressional charter to be an adviser to the federal government and, upon its own initiative, to identify issues of medical care, research, and education. Dr. Harvey V. Fineberg is president of the Institute of Medicine.

The **National Research Council** was organized by the National Academy of Sciences in 1916 to associate the broad community of science and technology with the Academy's purposes of furthering knowledge and advising the federal government. Functioning in accordance with general policies determined by the Academy, the Council has become the principal operating agency of both the National Academy of Sciences and the National Academy of Engineering in providing services to the government, the public, and the scientific and engineering communities. The Council is administered jointly by both Academies and the Institute of Medicine. Dr. Ralph J. Cicerone and Dr. C. D. Mote, Jr., are chair and vice chair, respectively, of the National Research Council.

www.national-academies.org

COMMITTEE ON QUALITY MEASURES FOR THE HEALTHY PEOPLE LEADING HEALTH INDICATORS

STEVEN M. TEUTSCH (*Chair*), Chief Science Officer, Los Angeles County Department of Public Health, CA
KEVIN GRUMBACH, Professor and Chair, University of California, San Francisco, Department of Family and Community Medicine
ROMANA HASNAIN-WYNIA, Director, Addressing Disparities, Patient-Centered Outcomes Research Institute, Washington, DC
JEWEL MULLEN, Commissioner of Health, Connecticut Department of Health, Hartford
JOHN OSWALD, Adjunct Assistant Professor, School of Public Health, University of Minnesota, Minneapolis
R. GIBSON PARRISH, Independent Consultant, Public Health Informatics Institute, Decatur, GA
GREG RANDOLPH, Director, Center for Public Health Quality, and Professor of Pediatrics and Adjunct Professor of Public Health, University of North Carolina at Chapel Hill
PATRICK REMINGTON, Professor and Associate Dean for Public Health, School of Medicine and Public Health, University of Wisconsin–Madison
JANE E. SISK, Scholar in Residence, Institute of Medicine, Washington, DC
PIERRE VIGILANCE, Associate Dean for Public Health Practice and Associate Professor of Global Health, School of Public Health and Health Services, George Washington University, Washington, DC

IOM Staff

ALINA BACIU, Study Director
ANDRÉS GAVIRIA, Research Associate
COLIN F. FINK, Senior Program Assistant
DORIS ROMERO, Financial Officer
HOPE HARE, Administrative Assistant
ROSE MARIE MARTINEZ, Director, Board on Population Health and Public Health Practice

Reviewers

This report has been reviewed in draft form by individuals chosen for their diverse perspectives and technical expertise, in accordance with procedures approved by the National Research Council's Report Review Committee. The purpose of this independent review is to provide candid and critical comments that will assist the institution in making its published report as sound as possible and to ensure that the report meets institutional standards of objectivity, evidence, and responsiveness to the study charge. The review comments and draft manuscript remain confidential to protect the integrity of the deliberative process. We thank the following individuals for their review of this report:

BECHARA CHOUCAIR, Chicago Department of Health
FERNANDO A. FERRER, University of Connecticut Health
    Center
MARTHE R. GOLD, City University of New York Medical School
KENNETH W. KIZER, Institute for Population Health
    Improvement
MARY PITTMAN, Public Health Institute
JOSHUA M. SHARFSTEIN, Maryland Department of Health and
    Mental Hygiene
SHOSHANA SOFAER, Baruch College of the City University of
    New York
JEANINE P. WIENER-KRONISH, Massachusetts General
    Hospital
MICHAEL WOLFSON, University of Ottawa
ALAN ZASLAVSKY, Harvard Medical School

   Although the reviewers listed above have provided many constructive comments and suggestions, they were not asked to endorse the conclusions or recommendations, nor did they see the final draft of the report before its release. The review of this report was overseen by **BOBBIE A. BERKOWITZ,** Columbia University, and **EDWARD B. PERRIN,** University of Washington. Appointed by the National Research Council and the Institute of Medicine, they were responsible for making certain that an independent examination of the report was carried out in accordance with institutional procedures and that all review comments were carefully considered. Responsibility for the final content of this report rests entirely with the authoring committee and the institution.

Contents

APPENDIXES

Summary

The Institute of Medicine (IOM) Committee on Quality Measures for the Healthy People Leading Health Indicators was charged by the Office of the Assistant Secretary for Health to identify measures of quality for the 12 Leading Health Indicator (LHI) topics and 26 LHIs in *Healthy People 2020*, the current version of the Department of Health and Human Services (HHS) 10-year agenda for improving the nation's health (see Box S-1 for the complete charge).

HHS referred the committee to two guiding documents: the *Consensus Statement of Quality in Public Health* (Public Health Quality Forum, 2008) and *Priority Areas for Improvement of Quality in Public Health* (Honoré and Scott, 2010). To respond to its charge, the committee reviewed these documents along with *Healthy People 2020* materials, earlier IOM reports, and reports of other organizations. The two documents provide a definition of quality in public health (see Box S-2); a list of nine quality aims, or "characteristics of quality in public health," and six priority areas, or drivers of quality improvement in the public health system, which are also part of the committee's charge. These quality characteristics and drivers for quality improvement are discussed in detail in Chapter 1.

The committee saw its task as helping to identify measures of quality to be used by partners in the health system broadly defined (beginning with public health and health care, plus contributions of other sectors) rather than identifying specific quality measures for specific public health programs. The former involves focusing primarily on intermediate and ultimate outcome measures, while identifying measures for specific programs requires a greater focus on process and intermediate outcomes.

BOX S-1
Statement of Task

A. Scope

The scope of work for this project is to use the nine aims for improvement of quality in public health (population-centered, equitable, proactive, health promoting, risk reducing, vigilant, transparent, effective, and efficient) as a framework to identify quality measures for the Healthy People Leading Health Indicators (LHIs).

B. Services to Be Performed

Task 1: A committee will review existing literature on the 12 LHI topics and the 26 Leading Health Indicators. Quality measures for the LHIs that are aligned with the nine aims for improvement of quality in public health will be identified. When appropriate, alignments with the six Priority Areas[a] for Improvement of Quality in Public Health will be noted in the Committee's report. The report should also address data reporting and analytical capacities that must be available to capture the measures and for demonstrating the value of the measures to improving population health.

Task 2: The committee will provide recommendations for how the measures can be used across sectors of the public health and health care systems.

---

[a] The six priority areas (also known as drivers) are population health metrics and information technology; evidence-based practices, research, and evaluation; systems thinking; sustainability and stewardship; policy; and workforce and education.

The purpose of measurement is threefold[1]: assessment, improvement, and accountability. A health department, for example, assesses health in its geographic area to inform community members and other stakeholders and to inform resource allocation. Health departments, hospitals, and other organizations use measures for improvement processes at different levels (e.g., ranging from program-specific efforts to system- or community-wide). Measures can also be used to demonstrate accountability to funders, partners, legislators, and communities.

---

[1] Some sources collapse two of the three.

BOX S-2
HHS Definition of Quality in Public Health

The HHS Public Health Quality Forum defined quality in public health as "the degree to which policies, programs, services and research for the population increase desired health outcomes and conditions in which the population can be healthy" (Public Health Quality Forum, 2008, p. 3).

The committee's charge called for using the nine aims or characteristics as a "framework to identify quality measures." The committee found that the nine quality characteristics in general do not directly lend themselves to being used as the framework for measures. The committee used as a conceptual framework the Health Outcome Logic Model (see Figure S-1), which is based on the structure–process–outcome framing of Donabedian (2005), but modified to reflect the definition of quality in public health provided in Box S-2. As high-level operating principles outlining the attributes of health systems (broadly defined) that seek to continuously improve quality, the nine characteristics relate primarily to the Resources and Characteristics component of the logic model.

The two smaller boxes on the left (Resources and Capacity and Interventions) align with the first two parts—structure and process, respectively—of the Donabedian framework, while the boxes in the middle and on the right (Healthy Conditions and Healthy Outcomes, respectively) refer to the third part of the Donabedian framework—outcomes, both intermediate and ultimate or long-term. Different types of metrics— referring to structure, process, and outcome—may be used as measures

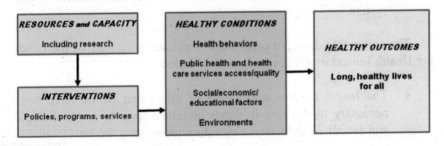

FIGURE S-1 Health outcome logic model.

of quality.[2] The committee focused on intermediate and ultimate outcomes because the measurements of Resources and Capacity do not directly link to the LHIs, while the specific process measures are numerous and reflect the Interventions actually implemented.

The committee used the logic model to help them classify the LHIs and to help select measures of quality related to the LHIs. For example, some of the LHIs, such as Air Quality Index (AQI), fit in the category of Healthy Conditions. The ultimate outcome related to AQI is lower cardiovascular and respiratory mortality and morbidity. Other LHIs, such as infant mortality, fit in the category Healthy Outcomes. Measures for Healthy Conditions related to infant mortality include prenatal care, childhood vaccines, and tobacco use.

The report outlines an approach to assist HHS in its efforts toward a national framework for quality that goes well beyond health care and clinical primary prevention. The approach, with three findings and six recommendations (see Box S-3, page 6), includes

1. The adoption of a logic model or conceptual framework to help identify loci for measures
2. The adoption of a set of recommended criteria to select measures of quality
3. A system to manage measures (to bring greater coherence and encourage parsimony and efficiency)
4. An entity to endorse measures of quality for the multisectoral health system
5. Consideration of potential uses for measures of quality by different partners and other contributors to the multisectoral health system

The committee does not offer a set of measures for each of the Leading Health Indicators for several reasons, including

- The length of time and extent of effort that would have been necessary to develop in-depth literature reviews for each topic and for all 26 indicators (including identifying the best available

---

[2] Two caveats: (1) Only outcome measures that are modifiable through some type of action or intervention can be used as measures of quality. Autism is one such example of a condition that does not yet have evidence-based preventive interventions. (2) It may be easier to describe quality measures for specific defined health care services (e.g., cancer screening), but harder to do so for the broad concept of population health.

evidence-based interventions for each), to develop a logic model for each LHI that would help identify measures related to each intervention, and to evaluate each measure according to standard, outlined criteria.

- The lasting value of developing a framework and process for a continually updated set of measures rather than identifying a static set of measures.

Furthermore, many measures of quality relate to the specific interventions implemented and are context specific. For this reason, too, describing a process seemed more useful than providing specific examples that would result from applying that process.

Because it focused on the 26 LHIs, the committee did not include other issues of great importance to the nation's health, such as disaster preparedness, the quality of the governmental public health system itself, and poverty as a health determinant. Pertinent to the last example, the *Healthy People 2020* chapter on social determinants was under development at the time the Secretary's Advisory Committee on National Health Promotion and Disease Prevention Objectives conducted its deliberations on the selection of the LHIs. Because of this, the social determinants of health are minimally reflected among the LHIs, but may warrant additional attention at this point in the process of implementing *Healthy People 2020* (e.g., consideration for adding to the LHIs). The committee also recognizes that the top health indicators at the local level may differ— suicide (a Healthy People LHI) may be a challenge in one community, while hepatitis C infection rates (not a Healthy People LHI) may be a priority concern in another. This is one of the reasons that the committee outlined criteria to be used by different communities to find measures that meet their needs.

Given the fast track nature of the committee's work, the committee conducted a literature review sufficient to enable it to provide a general discussion of potential quality measures for each of the 26 LHIs, with some examples provided in Table 3-1. Furthermore, the committee used LHIs under four topics (tobacco use; maternal, infant, and child health; environmental quality; and nutrition, physical activity, and obesity) to develop case studies building on the Health Outcome Logic Model to show the locus for potential measures at each step along the pathway to the relevant outcome. The committee thus offers a starter set toward a portfolio of measures of quality for the health system. The discussion preceding the four case studies also included an examination of the six priorities or drivers, and where appropriate, the ways in which planners and evaluators can reflect on the nine quality aims or characteristics in the process of selecting measures for use.

Finally, the committee discussed the relevance of quality measures to a variety of potential users, and the need and opportunities for a level of integration of services, research, data collection, and planning, as appropriate, between public health agencies and health care delivery organizations, with the goal of improving health outcomes. The committee viewed HHS's adoption of the Three-Part Aim (better care, lower cost,[3] and a healthier population) as creating a bridge between the health care and public health sectors or a platform for beginning to speak the same language and use some of the same metrics. Logic models similar to the one used in this report and the detailed models prepared for the four case studies can be used to explore resources, capacities, and interventions, especially at the local level, and to identify loci for measures, using the selection criteria to meet local needs. In closing, the committee offers suggestions for how measures of quality related to LHIs and, more broadly, for population health, could be used by decision makers, including government agencies, funders, hospitals and other health care organizations, and communities.

BOX S-3
Findings and Recommendations

Recommendation 1-1: The committee recommends that all partners in the multisectoral health system (public health, health care, community organizations, and others, as appropriate) should adopt as their explicit purpose to continually improve health outcomes of the entire population and the conditions in which people can be healthy. The extent to which this purpose is achieved reflects the overall quality of the health system.

Finding 2-1: The committee finds that partners in the multisectoral health system currently use a vast and complex array of measures of quality in a manner that seems uncoordinated.

Recommendation 2-1: The committee recommends that HHS and its partners in population health improvement (e.g., public health agencies, health care organizations, community organizations) adopt a portfolio of measures of the quality of the multisectoral health system. The portfolio of measures should

---

[3] The committee recognizes that the underlying goal with respect to cost is to control the increase in cost, and not necessarily reduce cost, as that is likely to be unfeasible.

   a.   include summary scores reflecting population-level healthy outcomes and healthy conditions;

   b.   balance parsimony with sufficient breadth; and

   c.   inform assessment, improvement, and accountability of the multisectoral health system.

Recommendation 2-2: The committee recommends that HHS and other relevant organizations adopt the following set of criteria for selecting and prioritizing measures of quality for use in population health improvement, including the Leading Health Indicators:

    Criteria for conditions or outcomes to be measured
    a.   Reflective of a high preventable burden[a]
    b.   Actionable at the appropriate level for intervention

    Criteria for the measures
    c.   Timely
    d.   Usable for assessing various populations
    e.   Understandable
    f.   Methodologically rigorous
    g.   Accepted and harmonized

Recommendation 2-3: The committee recommends HHS should ensure the implementation of a systematic approach to develop and manage a portfolio of measures of quality for the multisectoral health system. HHS also should establish or designate a nongovernmental and appropriately equipped entity to endorse measures of quality.

Recommendation 2-4: The committee recommends HHS should develop, implement, and support data collection, analysis, and dissemination mechanisms and infrastructure for the portfolio of quality measures so they are usable for health assessment and improvement at the national, state, and local levels.

Finding 3-1: The committee finds that

   a. Many of the LHIs are measures of health outcomes or of conditions that can directly affect health outcomes and are, therefore, measures of the quality of the multisectoral health system.[b]

   b. The LHIs that meet the definition above of a quality measure can be used for assessment, improvement, and accountability. To be used thus, they must be relevant and measurable at the national, state, and local levels.

   c. The LHIs reflect conditions or outcomes that directly contribute to the *Healthy People 2020* foundation measures (e.g., general health status, health-related quality of life) and the ecologic model[c] that underlies it, even if these are not explicitly represented among the LHIs.

continued

BOX S-3 Continued

Finding 4-1: The committee finds that the concept of a Three-Part Aim described in the National Quality Strategy could play a growing and important role in the process of establishing population health as an essential area of focus in transforming health care and health in the United States. The committee also finds that additional development is needed by users of the Three-Part Aim to incorporate evidence-based measures representing social and environmental determinants of health, equity, and the concept of total population health.

Recommendation 4-1: The committee recommends that HHS convene stakeholders to facilitate the use of measures of quality for the multisectoral health system and their integration into all activities under the Three-Part Aim with a special focus on the social and environmental determinants, equity, and the concept of total population health.

---

[a] The concept of high preventable burden has two components: high burden and existence of effective interventions. This concept (burden × effectiveness), refers to burden as the absolute burden, not relative burden. In other words, a condition like phenylketonuria (PKU) has a high preventable burden if one thinks of the denominator as all people with PKU, but it is a low absolute preventable burden if one uses the entire population.

[b] To illustrate, the rate of adult tobacco use is an LHI, but it can be used as a measure of quality because it gives an indication of the system's success in implementing evidence-based interventions to reduce use of tobacco. A rate of tobacco use that stagnates could provide an indication of a system that requires attention (an influx of resources, technical assistance in the area of policy analysis and development, collaboration, etc.) to improve its performance on reducing tobacco use.

[c] The ecological model is a diagram adapted from Whitehead and Dahlgren (1991) by an IOM committee and in *Healthy People 2020* planning by HHS to show the array of determinants of health, or the ecology of health as several concentric circles, beginning with individual level factors at the center (biologic and genetic factors); followed by behavior, family, social networks, and communities; followed by broad policies pertaining to the determinants of health (education, income, etc.) at the state and national level (see HHS, 2008; IOM, 2003a).

1

Introduction and Context

This chapter provides a discussion of terminology, a description of the context for the committee's charge (e.g., *Healthy People 2020* and the Affordable Care Act), and an outline of key milestones in the history of quality improvement theory and action in public health and health care.

TERMINOLOGY AND DEFINITIONS

The language of quality improvement in health care and public health presented the committee with its first challenge. Recognizing that the various concepts and terminology used to refer to quality are not standardized, a situation that leads to some confusion and a lack of precision (see, for example, discussion by Derose et al., 2002; Randolph et al., 2009), the committee sought to use terms consistently in its report (see glossary in Appendix A). Quality in public health has been defined as "the degree to which policies, programs, services and research for the population increase desired health outcomes and conditions in which the population can be healthy" (Public Health Quality Forum, 2008). Although the Department of Health and Human Services (HHS) documents on public health quality do not explicitly define quality measures, Derose and colleagues (2002) defined them as "quantitative statements about the capacity (structure), actions (processes), or results (outcomes) of public health practices" (p. 2).[1] Similarly, the National Quality Forum (NQF),

---

[1] Derose et al. (2002) use the term "quality indicators" and the committee considers the terms measures and indicators interchangeable in the context of this report. Also, while recognizing that quality and performance are distinct concepts, the committee finds that the term "performance measures" may be interchangeable with "quality measures." Unfortunately, none of the possible sources consulted, including materials from federal

which manages its Quality Positioning System for the health care delivery sector, describes its work as "evaluat[ing] and endors[ing] tools for standardized performance measurement, including: performance measures that assess structure, process, outcomes, and patient perceptions of care" (NQF, 2013). A cursory review of the 688 measures in the NQF system reveals a great range: some are measures of outcome (e.g., prevalence of adult tobacco use in the population), while others are more process-oriented (e.g., screening male smokers 65 through 75 years old for abdominal aortic aneurysm). Both definitions of measure provided above reflect the Donabedian framework of quality that has been widely used in health care quality improvement and that has also guided the committee in its development of a conceptual framing or logic model for this report. The definitions also suggest that different kinds of measures may be used in the work of quality improvement—measures of structure, process, and outcomes—and all these may be considered measures of quality.

Measuring and improving quality is a central focus in the health care delivery sector and in the implementation of the Affordable Care Act. However, the issue of quality is relevant to a far broader community of public- and private-sector contributors to the health of the population. Previous Institute of Medicine (IOM) reports have defined the multisectoral health system to include health care organizations (such as hospitals), state and local public health agencies, the education sector (e.g., schools and colleges), business, social services and other community-based organizations, faith-based groups, and many others (IOM, 2003a, 2011a, 2012). This report uses that broad definition of the health system.

The committee used the HHS definition of quality in public health (see Box S-2), with one modification—changing "quality in public health" (i.e., referring to the governmental public health agencies charged with protecting and promoting health in communities) to "quality in the multisectoral health system." Although the committee recognized that the public health quality work in HHS's Office of the Assistant Secretary for Health (OASH) is grounded in the activities of public health practice, the scope of the Leading Health Indicators (LHIs) (i.e., the inclusion of high school graduation and air quality measures), and the recognition that health is the result of multiple determinants and the ef-

---

agencies and from other organizations, shed light on how to distinguish quality and performance. The only obvious difference is that quality refers to a state of being, and performance refers to action, thus, measures of the state of being vs. measures of how well we do what we do (often incorporating attention to cost and efficiency). The committee found that delving more deeply into the language issue was not a productive endeavor.

forts of multiple actors and sectors (also reflected in the *Healthy People 2020* chapter on social determinants) makes it necessary to use a more expansive term. Thus, the committee refers to its work as identifying measures of quality for the multisectoral health system, in reference to the multiple contributors to improving health described above.

The more expansive description of the system is supported by comments made by the assistant secretary for health. In giving the committee its charge, he averred that the interface between clinical care and public health is an absolutely crucial arena for identifying and implementing measures of quality.

We are now in a time in the history of our country where we are really joining the worlds of health care and population health. We are joining the worlds of the clinic and the community. We are integrating what happens to people inside of a health care setting to what happens to people outside of a health care setting in the community. And that is where the future of all discussions about public health should lead.[2]

Although the health care delivery system is increasingly focused on population health, the committee found that focus reflects a relatively narrow interpretation of the term—population as the patient panel or group of covered lives (i.e., individuals insured). The committee preferred the Jacobson and Teutsch (2012) definition of total population health as the health of all persons living in a specified geopolitical area—a definition consistent with the history of public health practice.

In a further elaboration on what is meant by quality, the HHS Public Health Quality Forum outlined the nine *aims* for improvement of quality in public health, which are also described as *characteristics* of quality in the public health system. The characteristics are population-centered, equitable, proactive, health-promoting, risk-reducing, vigilant, transparent, effective, and efficient. The committee found the term "characteristics" more clear, and refers to "quality characteristics" in the report. The Public Health Quality Forum defined the characteristics in the following way:

---

[2] First meeting of the IOM Committee on Quality Measures for the Healthy People Leading Health Indicators, December 3, 2012, at the National Academy of Sciences Building, Washington, DC.

1. Population-centered—protecting and promoting healthy conditions and the health for the entire population
2. Equitable—working to achieve health equity
3. Proactive—formulating policies and sustainable practices in a timely manner, while mobilizing rapidly to address new and emerging threats and vulnerabilities
4. Health-promoting—ensuring policies and strategies that advance safe practices by providers and the population and increase the probability of positive health behaviors and outcomes
5. Risk-reducing—diminishing adverse environmental and social events by implementing policies and strategies to reduce the probability of preventable injuries and illness or other negative outcomes
6. Vigilant—intensifying practices and enacting policies to support enhancements to surveillance activities (e.g., technology, standardization, systems thinking/modeling)
7. Transparent—ensuring openness in the delivery of services and practices with particular emphasis on valid, reliable, accessible, timely, and meaningful data that is readily available to stakeholders, including the public
8. Effective—justifying investments by utilizing evidence, science, and best practices to achieve optimal results in areas of greatest need
9. Efficient—understanding costs and benefits of public health interventions and to facilitate the optimal utilization of resources to achieve desired outcomes

In addition to being asked to identify measures of public health quality within the framework provided by the nine quality characteristics, the committee was asked to comment on the relationship with the six priority areas, also described as drivers, for improvement of quality in public health. These are population health metrics and information technology; evidence-based practices, research, and evaluation; systems thinking; sustainability and stewardship; policy; and public health workforce and education.

CONTEXT

The OASH has spearheaded a national collaborative effort to develop a framework for quality in public health that complements ongoing efforts on health care quality, and fits into the larger context of

- Health care reform and the National Quality Strategy, the National Priorities Partnership, the National Prevention Strategy (National Priorities Partnership, 2011; NQF, 2012a).
- Major reports relevant to the nation's paradox of rising health care costs and poor outcomes (IOM, 2012; Stremikis et al., 2011).[3] A growing awareness of the evidence that determinants of health beyond genes, behavior, and health care play an important role in shaping the health of individuals and communities (reflected in the addition of a Social Determinants topic to *Healthy People 2020*).
- The history of standard setting, performance measurement, and quality improvement in public health, as attested to by the National Public Health Performance Standards, the Turning Point Performance Management National Excellence Collaborative, and more recently, the Multi-State Learning Collaborative associated with the voluntary national accreditation effort led by the Public Health Accreditation Board (Riley et al., 2010).
- Increased availability and use of health indicators, with key examples found in the decades-long national Healthy People effort, the state-oriented America's Health Rankings and the locally-focused County Health Rankings (IOM, 2011a; Remington and Booske, 2011; United Health Foundation, 2012). A more detailed overview of *Healthy People 2020* is provided below.

Healthy People 2020

Healthy People 2020 is a comprehensive set of national objectives for "improving the health of all Americans" and it is the most current version of a long-standing decennial HHS health planning effort. *Healthy People 2020* contains 42 topic areas, close to 600 objectives (with additional objectives under development), and 1,200 measures. The Leading Health Indicators represent a "smaller set of *Healthy People 2020* objectives," which "has been selected to communicate high-priority health issues and actions that can be taken to address them" (HHS, 2013).

---

[3] Studies published at the time of this writing in May 2013 indicated a slowdown in health care spending (Cutler and Sahni, 2013; Ryu et al., 2013)

Although *Healthy People 2020* does not explicitly refer to quality, quality in the performance of all partners in the multisectoral system is crucial to achieving desired health outcomes, for example, good schools to support students through graduation, effective health care delivery organizations that provide patient-centered medical homes, and effective public health agencies that serve as knowledge enterprises and help to convene stakeholders around health improvement.

The social determinants of health have been formally incorporated into *Healthy People 2020*. Koh and colleagues (2011) describe how the social determinants approach informed the Secretary's Advisory Committee on National Health Promotion and Disease Prevention Objectives for 2020 and informed the new social determinants topic in *Healthy People 2020*. The explicit recognition of multiple non-health factors at work in influencing health outcomes opens the door to a wider array of stakeholders. Given this context, the committee's view is that measures of quality related to the LHIs need not be limited to those outcomes and interventions over which governmental public health departments have direct responsibility or influence. Achieving the Healthy People objectives, and the overarching, aspirational goal of long, healthy lives for all people in the United States clearly requires collaboration with other sectors, within and outside government, and at all geographic levels. Although the nine quality characteristics refer primarily to the governmental public health agencies, it is well understood that public health action is not limited to government, therefore the committee considers the findings and recommendations in this report relevant to partners in health care delivery and in other sectors.

In its survey of measures related to the LHIs (see Box 1-1), the committee noted that many such measures are found in the health care delivery system or in an area of overlap between public health and health care. Changes precipitated by the Affordable Care Act also offer opportunities for health care to expand its role well beyond the patient care, and for public health and health care to work together in new ways. One such example is the expansion of concepts of community benefit offered by tax-exempt hospitals to include community-building activities and collaboration with other sectors in improving the health of the community in a more holistic manner than solely through the patient–provider interaction.

BOX 1-1
Healthy People 2020 **Leading Health Indicator Topics
and Leading Health Indicators**

1. **Access to Health Services**
   1) Persons with medical insurance (AHS-1.1)
   2) Persons with a usual primary care provider (AHS-3)
2. **Clinical Preventive Services**
   3) Adults who receive a colorectal cancer screening based on the most recent guidelines (C-16)
   4) Adults with hypertension whose blood pressure is under control (HDS-12)
   5) Adult diabetic population with an [hemoglobin] A1c value greater than 9 percent (D-5.1)
   6) Children aged 19 to 35 months who receive the recommended doses of DTaP, polio, MMR, Hib, hepatitis B, varicella, and PCV vaccines (IID-8)
3. **Environmental Quality**
   7) Air Quality Index (AQI) exceeding 100 (EH-1)
   8) Children aged 3 to 11 years exposed to secondhand smoke (TU-11.1)
4. **Injury and Violence**
   9) Fatal injuries (IVP-1.1)
   10) Homicides (IVP-29)
5. **Maternal, Infant, and Child Health**
   11) Infant deaths (MICH-1.3)
   12) Preterm births (MICH-9.1)
6. **Mental Health**
   13) Suicides (MHMD-1)
   14) Adolescents who experience major depressive episodes (MDEs) (MHMD-4.1)
7. **Nutrition, Physical Activity, and Obesity**
   15) Adults who meet current Federal physical activity guidelines for aerobic physical activity and muscle strengthening activity (PA-2.4)
   16) Adults who are obese (NWS-9)
   17) Children and adolescents who are considered obese (NWS-10.4)
   18) Total vegetable intake for persons aged 2 years and older (NWS-15.1)
8. **Oral Health**
   19) Persons aged 2 years and older who used the oral health care system in past 12 months (OH-7)
9. **Reproductive and Sexual Health**
   20) Sexually active females aged 15 to 44 years who received reproductive health services in the past 12 months (FP-7.1)
   21) Persons living with HIV who know their serostatus (HIV-13)

continued

BOX 1-1 Continued

10. Social Determinants
    22) Students who graduate with a regular diploma 4 years after starting 9th grade (AH-5.1)
11. Substance Abuse
    23) Adolescents (12-17 years old) using alcohol or any illicit drugs during the past 30 days (SA-13.1)
    24) Adults engaging in binge drinking during the past 30 days (SA-14.3)
12. Tobacco
    25) Adults who are current cigarette smokers (TU-1.1)
    26) Adolescents who smoked cigarettes in the past 30 days (TU-2.2)

NOTES: AH = adolescent health; AHS = access to health services; C = cancer; D = diabetes; EH = environmental health; FP = family planning; HDS = heart disease and stroke; HIV = human immunodeficiency virus; IID = immunization and infectious diseases; IVP = injury and violence prevention; MHMD = mental health and mental disorders; MICH = maternal, infant, and child health; NWS = nutrition and weight status; OH = oral health; PA = physical activity; SA = substance abuse; TU = tobacco use.

A SHORT HISTORY OF QUALITY IN HEALTH CARE AND PUBLIC HEALTH

The notion of monitoring and reporting quality in health care is very familiar and well explored. The public health field also has a history of quality improvement initiatives. The Institute of Medicine began its examination of quality in health care soon after its 1970 founding, with the 1974 report *Advancing the Quality of Health Care: A Policy Statement* (IOM, 1974), and IOM's work in this area has continued through many influential reports, most notably *Crossing the Quality Chasm* (IOM, 2001). In parallel with the IOM work on quality in the late 1990s, the President established the Advisory Commission on Consumer Protection and Quality and Health Care in 1996, and that Commission released its report in 1998 (President's Advisory Commission on Consumer Protection and Quality in the Health Care Industry, 1998). On the public health side, the 1997 IOM report *Improving Health in the Community: The Role for Performance Monitoring* described the components of the community health improvement process, examined the role of performance monitoring in that process, and identified possible tools for communities wishing to develop performance measures.

In 1994, the IOM Council issued a white paper, "America's Health in Transition: Protecting and Improving Quality" (IOM, 1994), which included the following statement:

> Quality can and must be measured, monitored, and improved. Policymakers, whether in the public or the private sector at local, state, or federal levels, must insist that the tools for measuring and improving quality be applied. These approaches require constant modification and reassessment—that is, the continual development of new strategies and the refinement of old ones. Furthermore, credible, objective, and nonpolitical surveillance and reporting of quality in *health*[4] and health care must be explicitly articulated and vigorously applied as change takes place.

The current committee's work reflects on these ideas in several ways. First, the committee recognized that the topic of quality and quality improvement is complex, and that the concepts and terminology that operate in this realm of quality are not standardized or widely agreed on (see, for example, discussion in Derose et al., 2002; Randolph et al., 2009). Second, the phrases "reporting of quality in *health* and health care" reflect a distinction that is crucial when talking about quality, and that played an important role in the committee's deliberations. That is, measuring and improving quality does not apply only to the delivery of health care services, such as in eliminating overuse, underuse, and misuse of medical procedures. As described in *Improving Health in the Community* (IOM, 1997) and more recently, in *For the Public's Health: The Role of Measurement in Action and Accountability* (IOM, 2011a), measurement is essential for improving the health of the population outside the clinical setting—improving health in communities; it shines a light on the social and environmental factors that shape health outcomes (i.e., the determinants of health) and thus helps mobilize people and groups to take action to alter those factors. As recent public health quality efforts in HHS have emphasized, quality also refers to nine characteristics (listed above) that must be present in the delivery of population-based interventions, and more broadly, in implementing any interventions intended (or known) to improve the population's health. Third, in light of the 1988 definition of public health, that is, "fulfilling society's interest in assuring conditions in which people can be healthy," the committee believes that quality in the context of population health im-

---

[4] Italics added.

provement relates to all the systems (or their contributions) that create conditions that shape a community's health outcomes. Beyond health care and public health organizations, which are wholly dedicated to health-related goals, the sectors of education, transportation, housing, business, and planning are among those that contribute in different ways to health outcomes. High school graduation, for example, contributes to better health outcomes (Freudenberg and Ruglis, 2007), but is not a factor controlled by governmental public health agencies. Fourth, the committee reiterates the recommendation of the 2011 IOM report *For the Public's Health: The Role of Measurement in Action and Accountability,* which echoed others in the field (e.g., Brownson et al., 2010) in calling for measures of a community's intrinsic health in the sense of health-promoting or health-supporting features of a community, such as walkability, ample green and recreational space, quality housing, adequate healthful food sources, and an information environment that is shaped to support health (e.g., fast food restaurant advertising).

Several IOM reports on quality in health care have defined quality as "the degree to which health services for individuals and populations increase the likelihood of desired health outcomes and are consistent with current professional knowledge" (IOM, 1990, 1998, 1999). One of those reports explained that "viewed most broadly, the purpose of quality measurement [in health care] is to secure for Americans the most health care value for society's very large investment" (IOM, 1999, p. 2). These reports and the definitions and frameworks they have put forward, along with important work from the Institute for Healthcare Improvement and others in the field, have served as part of the foundation for the work of the HHS Public Health Quality Forum (PHQF). The PHQF, convened in 2008 to stimulate "a national movement for coordinated quality improvement efforts across all levels in the public health system" comprises the HHS Office of Public Health and Science, several HHS agencies (HHS, 2012), and also received input from several stakeholder organizations (Public Health Quality Forum, 2008). Building on the 1990 IOM definition, the PHQF defined quality in public health somewhat analogously as "the degree to which policies, programs, services, and research for the population increase desired health outcomes and conditions in which the population can be healthy" (Public Health Quality Forum, 2008). The concept of conditions links to the 1988 IOM report that defined public health, and also to the ever-expanding evidence base on the social and environmental determinants of health. The committee's charge places its work at the intersection of the *Healthy People 2020* population health measurement effort and the public health quality improvement effort. These two activities, which are both in the OASH, are linked because the ultimate evidence of quality in a system is demonstrated by measures showing good outcomes.

Almost a decade after the 1999 IOM report on quality in health care, HHS released the 2008 PHQF report *Consensus Statement on Quality in the Public Health System.* The statement built on the work of the 1998 report of the President's Commission on Consumer Protection and Quality in the Health Care Industry and the IOM report *Crossing the Quality Chasm,* which in 2001 described the six aims for improvement in quality of care: safe, timely, effective, efficient, equitable, and patient-centered (see Box 1-1).

Between 2008 and the writing of the present report, several important activities have been launched or conducted that further shape the field and inform the committee's work to identify quality measures for the 26 LHIs. In 2010, HHS was charged by the Affordable Care Act (ACA)[5] to develop a National Strategy for Quality Improvement in Health Care. In March 2011, HHS submitted the National Quality Strategy to Congress, followed in 2012 by the first *Annual Report to Congress* (Honore et al., 2011). A goal of the National Quality Strategy is to build consensus nationally on how to measure health care quality and align federal and state efforts "to reduce duplication and create efficiencies— not just in measurement but in quality improvement efforts as well" (National Priorities Partnership, 2011, pp. 1-3). The NQF convened more than 50 public and private organizations in the National Priorities Partnership which provides ongoing input on the implementation of the Strategy. The Strategy and the work of NQF were part of the committee's information gathering, as described elsewhere in the report. The National Quality Strategy also introduced a Three-Part Aim, modeled on the Triple Aim framework developed by the Institute for Healthcare Improvement in 2006, which called for improving the experience of care, improving the health of populations, and reducing per capita costs of health care. Similarly, the Three-Part Aim calls for

1. Better care: Improve the overall quality of care, by making health care more patient-centered, reliable, accessible, and safe.
2. Healthy people/healthy communities: Improve the health of the U.S. population by supporting proven interventions to address behavioral, social, and environmental determinants of health in addition to delivering higher-quality care.

---

[5] Section 3011.

   3. Affordable care: Reduce the cost of quality health care for individuals, families, employers, and government (HHS, 2012).

The second component of the Three-Part Aim clearly identifies a focus on the population as a whole (not merely subpopulations of patients covered by a specific insurer, or patients with a specific condition), consistent with public health theory and with earlier work in HHS.

Throughout its deliberations, the committee that produced this report used the logic model shown in Figure 1-1. The model is a simple illustration of the PHQF's definition of quality: "the degree to which policies, programs, services and research for the population increase desired health outcomes and conditions in which the population can be healthy." The model is obviously not intended to capture all the complete and complex pathways from inputs to outputs and outcomes that relate to health: it is intended instead to serve as a general guide for how to think about this complex area in the process of identifying measures of quality. The model, which resembles the logic model used by a previous IOM committee (see IOM, 2011a, 2012), shows system structure (Resources and Capacity) and processes (Interventions) on the far left. These influence Healthy Conditions (i.e., the determinants of health), which in turn lead to intermediate and ultimate population health outcomes. The logic model provides a framework for discussing and organizing the LHIs and measures of quality associated with them. The grouping of measures according to domains in a conceptual framework (i.e., logic model) was first used by the developers of the County Health Rankings, as a way to communicate the relationship between health outcomes, their determinants, and the programs and policies that can be used to improve population health (Remington and Booske, 2011).

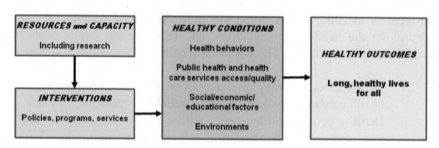

FIGURE 1-1 Health outcome logic model.

Viewed from left to right, the model shows concisely the relationship among system inputs and structure, processes, and outputs and outcomes. Resources and Capacity refers to the systems requirements such as funding, a trained and capable workforce, information technology capabilities, and the knowledge base: the six drivers of quality improvement in public health are found here. Research is especially important because it serves as a foundation for policies, programs, and services, which in turn lead to healthy conditions and yield healthy outcomes. In practical terms, identifying measures of quality requires an evidence base that allows one to identify which interventions used to achieve a specific outcome are effective and to determine the extent to which they are effective (magnitude of effect). Absent a strong research enterprise to inform the work of improving population health, the measurement of quality is seriously limited.

The committee discussed measures of quality in reference to the model, with measures including and related to the LHIs fitting largely under the Healthy Conditions (determinants of health and intermediate outcomes) and Healthy Outcomes headings. The committee focused on intermediate and ultimate outcomes because the specific process measures are too numerous and are dependent on the interventions actually implemented. Although the topic of health disparities is not explicitly identified in the logic model, the committee notes that inequities at the level of conditions that influence health are linked with disparities in health outcomes.

In response to the part of the charge requesting a discussion of alignment between the "the aims for improvement of quality in public health" (also known as "characteristics to guide public health practices") and the measures of quality, the committee found that the characteristics of quality cannot be conceptually aligned with specific measures, since they describe the system as a whole, and refer to the public health system or interventions rather than quality measures per se. For example, measures of quality cannot be classified as vigilant or effective, but they can provide information about the existence of interventions or system capacity that demonstrate vigilance and effectiveness. The presence of a surveillance system (a resource or capacity), for example, may provide indication that the system is vigilant and effective. The six drivers of quality improvement in public health—metrics and information technology; evidence-based practices, research, and evaluation; systems thinking; sustainability and stewardship; policy; and workforce and education—also fit under Resources and Capacity. This is discussed in more detail in Chapter 3. The Healthy Conditions segment of the model also serves as a link to the ecological model[6] describing the multiple determinants of health. An important caveat to consider in reviewing the logic model is that it is not intended to suggest a definitive classification system, but rather, a structured and coherent way to approach measurement of quality. The committee's deliberations about the model and contents showed that assigning an item to one of the boxes is not necessarily straightforward or able to garner universal agreement. The categorization of health care was one area that required extensive discussion, and the committee reached agreement that health care access and quality fit in the Healthy Conditions segment, while the programs, policies, and services that are needed to have high-quality health care conditions belong in the Interventions box on the left. As a specific example, mammography screening programs, tobacco cessation services, and community education programs about healthy eating would go under Interventions, while mammography screening rates (women screened for breast cancer), persons receiving tobacco cessation services, and the proportion of population informed about the value of healthy eating would be classified as Healthy Conditions. There are programs, policies, and services related to all of the Healthy Conditions in the logic model. For example, for socioeconomic status, the programs and policies could include per capita funding for education and earned income tax credits. Environmental conditions result from programs and policies such as zoning policies, bike path funding, and safe routes to school. Health care "conditions" are a result of such policies and programs as health care reform, funding for community health centers, employer mandates, and clean air policies (i.e., to prevent asthma attacks in vulnerable groups). Health behaviors are influenced by such policies as drunk driving laws, seat belt laws, minimum purchase laws, and smoking bans.

Although Resources and Capacity is part of the logic model, the committee's examination of measures of inputs was limited. One reason for this is the fact that these types of measures are more specific to the interventions selected and this level of detail is beyond the scope of a report such as this. Ongoing efforts exist to measure or verify aspects of a system that could contribute to making it high-performing (see IOM,

---

[6] The ecological model is a diagram adapted from Whitehead and Dahlgren (1991) and used by IOM committees and HHS to show the array of determinants of health, or the ecology of health, beginning with individual level factors at the center (biology/genetics), then on to behavior, family, social networks, and communities, followed by broad policies pertaining to the determinants of health (education, income, etc.) at the state and national level (see HHS, 2013, and IOM, 2003a, p. 52).

2011a, for examples). The voluntary national effort of public health accreditation is one such effort (Public Health Accreditation Board, 2011).

The model can be used for several purposes. First, it illustrates the main steps in a process of health improvement: attention to resources and capacities, implementing interventions that work, achievement of intermediate outcomes (e.g., improvement in the conditions that influence health), and ultimate outcomes. Second, it helps illustrate that the quality characteristics (population-centered, equitable, proactive, health-promoting, risk-reducing, vigilant, transparent, effective, and efficient) refer to capacities and interventions, not to outcomes. For example, a health department with a robust injury surveillance system is demonstrating the quality characteristic "vigilant." Regular reporting (e.g., annual) about a community unintentional injury data demonstrates "transparent." Having the capacity to implement and then actually implementing evidence-based interventions to reduce injury in the community demonstrates a health department is population-centered and risk-reducing. Third, the logic model could be used to illustrate the relationships among different types of measures (as shown in the detailed logic models in Chapter 3). Fourth, the logic model can also inform thinking about the usefulness (e.g., applicability) and feasibility (e.g., availability of necessary data) of various kinds of measures at different levels of action—national, state, and local.

Under ideal circumstances the achievement of the highest possible health-related outcomes may be considered the ultimate indicator of a high-quality health (not health care) system. In practice, things are considerably more complex, both because of the lack of a singular sector or entity with the responsibility and the ability to improve the health of a population and because of the vast array of factors that influence health (e.g., the likelihood that a neighborhood with a very high socioeconomic level will have superior health outcomes by virtue of that fundamental characteristic, regardless of the presence of a competent health care delivery system or public health agency). One measure of health—life expectancy—has been tracked for a long time and is perhaps the most universally understood indicator of a nation's health status.

Although they are not explicitly reflected in the LHIs, the foundation health measures of *Healthy People 2020* reside in four domains:

1. General health status (life expectancy, healthy life expectancy, years of potential life lost; physically and mentally unhealthy days; self-assessed health status; limitation of activity; chronic disease prevalence);

2. Health-related quality of life and well-being (measures of physical, mental, and social health-related quality of life; well-being and satisfaction; participation in common activities);
3. Determinants of health (biology, genetics, individual behavior, access to health services, and the environment in which people are born, live, learn, play, work, and age); and
4. Disparities (measures of differences in health status associated with race and ethnicity, gender, physical and mental ability, and geography) (HHS, 2012).

Healthy People 2020's overarching goals—longer, healthier lives; health equity; health-promoting environments for all; and the promotion of healthy life, development, and behaviors across the lifespan—acknowledge the importance of looking to population health outcomes to gauge the nation's progress in meeting health objectives (HHS, 2008; Koh, 2010).

In a context of rapidly proliferating, duplicative, overlapping, and imperfect measures, the committee envisions a multisectoral health system in which

- All participant organizations define the quality of the system in terms of progress toward "long, healthy lives for all."
- All participant organizations assess quality in the multisectoral health system via a well-constructed portfolio of measures spanning the resources available, the interventions (programs, policies, etc.), the conditions in which people live (referring broadly to all the determinants of health including behavior and the social environment), and the health outcomes (see Figure 1-1; see Recommendation 2-1 for the description of a well-constructed portfolio).
- Communities report about their overall public health quality annually and use specific measures regularly for the purpose of improving outcomes.

The committee reviewed the IOM report *Crossing the Quality Chasm* (2001) and its recommendation made to all components of the health care delivery system. In the same spirit of mobilizing partners around improving quality, the present committee makes an analogous recommendation pertaining to quality in the health system writ large.

RECOMMENDATION 1-1: **All partners in the multi-sectoral health system should adopt as their explicit purpose to continually improve health outcomes of the entire population and the conditions in which people can be healthy. The extent to which this purpose is achieved reflects the overall quality of the health system.**

To help in achieving this recommendation, this report outlines selection criteria and provides sample metrics to support HHS and its partners in enhancing quality to ultimately improve population health.

The intersection of quality improvement and the *Healthy People 2020* effort in HHS, against the backdrop of health care reform and growing interest in population health concepts make this a time of great opportunity to create platforms on which public health and health care can begin to use same language, employ some of the same metrics, and work together to bring about the shared goal of long, healthy lives for all.

2

Criteria for Selecting Measures

The committee was asked to describe methods for selecting quality measures for the Leading Health Indicators (LHIs) and for the work of improving the public's health more broadly. In this chapter, the committee offers guidance for selecting measures to assess and improve quality in the multisectoral health system, and especially among health care and public health participants.

To make progress toward long, healthy lives for all, pertinent stakeholders need to create healthy communities and address the underlying factors that influence health outcomes and disparities in those outcomes among different subgroups. Measurement is an essential ingredient of such efforts. The committee believes that a summary measure of population health is needed along with or as a part of a set of measures of quality. Such a measure is needed for every community and must be consistently defined in order for public health officials and members of the public to understand the quality of their public health system and to compare it with national and other appropriate benchmarks of quality (e.g., summary scores measuring system quality for peer counties or states and for the nation), and to support mutual accountability among partners and contributors in the multisectoral health system. The committee reviewed the 2011 Institute of Medicine (IOM) report *For the Public's Health: The Role of Measurement in Action and Accountability* and endorses its rationale and recommendation for the national adoption of a summary measure of population health equivalent to health-adjusted life years (HALYs) or health-adjusted life expectancy (HALE) (IOM, 2011a).

It is incumbent on decision makers and professionals working in quality improvement to consistently answer the question "Quality for whom?" Furthermore, once this question is answered, the public health agencies and the health care delivery organizations need policies to translate into action the broad goal of addressing disparities in health status. It is not enough to monitor and report disparities; measurement can also serve as a tool to ascertain whether inputs (e.g., resources and capacity) and processes (e.g., policies, programs, and services) are succeeding in moving health improvement efforts toward the desired health outcomes and greater equity. Equity across all groups by age, socioeconomic status, race, gender, and sexual orientation can be measured as ranges (i.e., differences among groups), and using such metrics as the Gini coefficient, the index of dissimilarity, the slope index of inequality, and the index of disparity developed for *Healthy People 2010* (Pearcy and Keppel, 2002). It is possible to publish health-adjusted life expectancy data by quintiles of income, sex, race, and ethnicity (see, for example, the evidence reviewed by Clarke et al. [2010]). One strategy for ensuring that equity is a guiding principle from the beginning is to apply a consistent and scientifically justifiable approach to race/ethnicity and socioeconomic classification in the process of population measurement. Also, it is not enough to look at descriptive data; rather, it is important that system inputs be used to drive improvement in achieving equitable outcomes. Asada and colleagues (2013) have proposed a potentially useful analytic approach to measuring disparities, using functional limitation data (i.e., activities of daily living) from the 2009 American Community Survey to develop disparity profiles by states, showing whether disparities were associated primarily with race and ethnicity, socioeconomic factors, or both. Because the social determinants chapter in *Healthy People 2020* was under development during the deliberations leading to selection of the LHIs, those factors are minimally reflected in the LHIs. Although it is beyond this report's scope to discuss the social determinants of health in depth, measuring the inequities (in inputs) that lead to disparities in outcome provides essential information about systemic challenges or obstacles at the level of government policy and institutional practices (see, for example, the IOM [2003c] report *Unequal Treatment: Confronting Racial and Ethnic Disparities in Health Care*).

The committee attempted to apply a coherence-creating, unifying, standardized quality measurement approach to the LHIs, but the LHIs were not designed primarily from a quality perspective. The final selection of LHIs for *Healthy People 2020* was made by HHS with input from the IOM (2011b)[1] and the Secretary's Advisory Committee on Health

---

[1] The IOM's 2011 report *Leading Health Indicators for Healthy People 2020: Letter Report* does provide that report's authoring committee's rationale for selecting candidate LHIs for HHS (IOM, 2011b).

Promotion and Disease Prevention (Honore et al., 2011). The present IOM committee recognizes that HHS and its advisers had to reconcile many considerations in a complex process that included considering the burden of disease; managing mandates, resources, current priorities, and capabilities; weighing and balancing stakeholder interests and expectations; and making important tradeoffs. This array of factors and forces explains both the very large and heterogeneous set of *Healthy People 2020* objectives (approximately 1,200 that cover many but not necessarily all top burden of disease priorities) and the heterogeneity or dissimilarity of the LHIs (population vs. clinical/individual, disease specific vs. risk behavior, related to one outcome/endpoint vs. pertinent to a dozen outcomes/endpoints), which presented a challenge to the IOM committee in its attempt to identify a coherent set of quality measures.

There were also some constraints on the HHS advisory committee's work. For example, one requirement was that the LHIs be drawn from the *Healthy People 2020* objectives. As a result of the many considerations and constraints made in selecting them, the resulting set of 26 LHIs (see Box 1-1 for the complete list of LHIs) is highly heterogeneous: some LHIs relate to outcomes, while others relate to processes. Four of the LHIs—fatal injuries, homicides, infant deaths, and suicides—are themselves outcome measures. Another four are intermediate outcome measures (preterm births, adolescents with major depressive episodes, adults with controlled hypertension, and adult diabetics with poor glucose control) and 12 LHIs could be classified as measures of the effectiveness of an intervention.

When the LHIs are organized according to the logic model above, most measures fit in the categories of Healthy Conditions and Health Outcomes. Few LHIs fit in the category of Interventions (one example is receiving primary care services), and none fits under Resources and Capacity. Despite the lack of LHIs in this last category, measures in this area are an important contributor to a system's success in moving toward desired outcomes. For example, research exploring the relationship between public health funding and outcomes is still in its early stages, but Mays and Smith (2011) have provided suggestive evidence that public health funding is correlated with better health outcomes. Some aspects of Resources and Capacity were discussed in a previous IOM report (2012), and reviewing that report's discussion of the "foundational capabilities" of public health agencies shows a great deal of congruence with the six drivers of quality improvement in public health.

The committee did not set out to replicate the many causal networks that could be developed to show how various system inputs lead to cer-

tain intermediate outcomes that result in ultimate population health outcomes. This has been done by others for various chronic diseases, including the Centers for Disease Control and Prevention (CDC)/
National Institutes of Health (NIH) Prevention Impacts Simulation Model (PRISM) described in Homer and colleagues (2010) and also the work
of Jones and colleagues (2006), and Wolfson and Rowe (2001), and although many of the models available have specific purposes and limitations, they illustrate the complexity of causal factors and the interactions
among them. They also suggest important methods for structuring and
understanding the relationship of specific interventions to specific health
outcomes, and they help quantify components and indicate which interventions might be best in a specific place to achieve a desired set of outcomes. A previous IOM committee called for modeling to help inform
decision makers about interventions that are likely to have the greatest
impact (IOM, 2011a). That committee recommended "that the Department of Health and Human Services (HHS) coordinate the development
and evaluation and advance the use of predictive and system-based simulation models to understand the health and consequences of underlying
determinants of health. HHS should also use modeling to assess intended
and unintended outcomes associated with policy, funding, investment,
and resource options" (IOM, 2011a, p. 103 [Recommendation 6]). Such
work would also help identify, develop, and refine measures of quality. In
Chapter 3 (see Table 3-1), the committee offers sample measures along the
trajectory of the various LHIs. For example, the update of childhood vaccines
is an intermediate outcome, whose ultimate outcomes are the rates of morbidity and mortality from certain infectious diseases.

GENERAL CONSIDERATIONS FOR SELECTING AND
PRESENTING MEASURES OF QUALITY

The committee provides some preliminary considerations for selecting measures of quality related to the LHIs and for population health
more broadly. Also, as previously noted, the quality characteristics do
not apply directly to the LHIs or to measures of quality. Measures cannot
in and of themselves be thought of as effective, population-centered, or
transparent. However, several of the characteristics are embedded in the
criteria for measure selection as described below. Measures of quality
may measure outcomes or intermediate outcomes, may reflect on effi-

ciency or on cost-effectiveness[2] and will ideally be associated with evidence-based interventions (e.g., programs and policies).

In its deliberations, the committee agreed that although measures of quality may be presented as long lists or catalogues (similar to the National Quality Forum–endorsed system of almost 700 measures, or as an extension of the 1,200 *Healthy People 2020* objectives themselves), a set or portfolio of measures is likely to be more useful to—and thus, more used by—practitioners involved in quality improvement, and also more informative to communities and other audiences wishing to understand how the system is performing. There are at least two such comprehensive, but parsimonious, measure portfolios currently in use: America's Health Rankings (AHR), which uses 44 measures, and the County Health Rankings (CHR), which uses 30 measures in 5 domains (Remington and Booske, 2011). The AHR has been published since 1990 (United Health Foundation, 2012) and represents an effort to quantify and analyze the status and changes in health in the U.S. population from year to year. The information used is from publicly accessible data, collected mostly by the federal government. A major data source is Behavioral Risk Factor Surveillance System (BRFSS) of the Centers for Disease Control and Prevention (CDC), but it has limited usefulness at the local level. AHR reports the rankings by state and includes sections on health disparities and how the United States compares to other countries. More recently, CHR began rankings by county within each state. CHR is based at the University of Wisconsin Population Health Institute, which has ranked Wisconsin's counties since 2003. CHR uses data from publicly available local and federal government sources. Other pertinent measurement activities include the CDC Community Health Status Indicators, which provides a portfolio of 200 measures, with a set for each of the 3,141 U.S. counties, and allows comparisons between peer counties to inform quality improvement efforts and the sharing of best practices. The 2011 IOM report *For the Public's Health: The Role of Measurement in Action and Accountability* provides additional descriptions of indicator efforts. In the realm of health care delivery there also are multiple ongoing efforts, ranging from the National Committee on Quality Assurance HEDIS (Healthcare Effectiveness Data and Information Set) measures, to the hundreds of additional measures from many other organizations provided as part of the National Quality Forum's Quality Positioning System, its measure endorsement process. Finally, the Agency for

---

[2] The "extent to which the results are achieved at a lower cost compared with alternatives" (World Bank, 2007, p. 65).

Healthcare Research and Quality (ARHQ) National Quality Measures Clearinghouse contains a large collection of measures (more than 2,000)—the vast majority of measures belong to the health care delivery domain and small number are listed under the population health domain.[3]

CRITERIA FOR MEASURE SELECTION

In comments made at the committee's first meeting, the Assistant Secretary for Health suggested the committee provide methodological guidance that could be used in selecting measures of quality. In response, the committee reviewed a number of existing resources for sample criteria (see Table 2-1 below and Table B-1 in Appendix B for a description of criteria across several different sources). The committee's review included the National Quality Forum's criteria for evaluating measures, the Institute for Healthcare Improvement's key measurement principles that apply to the Triple Aim, the HHS Secretary's Advisory Committee on Health Promotion and Disease Prevention Objectives for 2020 operational criteria for selection of LHIs, the 2003 IOM report *Priority Areas for National Action: Transforming Health Care Quality* and the 2010 IOM report *Future Directions for the National Healthcare Quality and Disparities Reports*. The AHRQ National Quality Measures Clearinghouse (not in the table) provides the following criteria for measures included in their database: (1) the measure is cited in peer-reviewed/National Library of Medicine journal, (2) the measure has documented evidence of reliability and validity, and (3) the measure has been developed, adopted, adapted, or endorsed by an appropriate organization.[4]

With the exception of the criteria for selecting LHIs, the sets of criteria listed were developed for measures largely pertinent to health care delivery, and the committee did not feel that any existing set of measures was sufficiently specific for selecting measures of quality for the multisectoral health system. Because none of the sets of criteria listed is primarily oriented toward population health, they miss some of the nuances that are important in population health interventions. For example, data availability at the state and local level is a critical issue for population health measures, but not for clinical care measures, where data are intrinsically part of the medical record.

---

[3] The population health domain includes dimensions such as population health state, social determinants of health, and environment.
[4] See http://www.qualitymeasures.ahrq.gov/about/inclusion-criteria.aspx (accessed May 31, 2013).

Topically similar criteria in these sets were grouped into five categories: (1) impact or importance of the condition or outcome to be measured; (2) improvability, or the extent of the gap between current practice and evidence-based best practice and the likelihood that the gap can be closed; (3) scientific soundness of the measure, including validity and reliability; (4) geographic, temporal, and population coverage to ensure that the measure has sufficient granularity to be useful in monitoring actions to improve health at different geographic levels in important population subgroups; and (5) data availability to ensure that data are readily available in a form useful for quality and performance measurement (see Table 2-1 and Appendix B). The first two categories—impact and improvability—refer to characteristics of condition(s), outcome(s), and associated interventions that a measure would address, while the final three categories—scientific soundness, coverage, and data availability—address characteristics of the measures themselves. Thus, the committee developed a set of criteria that embody most characteristics of these existing sets, while using words and providing definitions that indicate characteristics that are more relevant for population health, and emphasizing certain criteria that are particularly important for population health, such as coverage at the state and local level, where many population-based interventions are implemented. The committee also recognizes the potential usefulness of a stepwise approach to applying

TABLE 2-1 Quick Comparison of Published Criteria for Measure Selection (Detailed Table Provided in Appendix B)

Category of Criteria	Published Criteria			
	NQF, 2012b	HHS SAC, 2011	IOM, 2010	IOM, 2003b
Impact (importance)	X	X	X	X
Improvability	X	unclear	X	X
Scientifically sound measure	X	n/a	X	n/a
Geographic, temporal, and population coverage	n/a	X	X	unclear
Data availability	X	n/a	X	n/a

NOTES: X indicates that the published criteria included one or more items in the category listed in the first column; n/a = not applicable.

these criteria, in which the target of potential measures is first evaluated for importance and improvability (seen through a population health lens), followed by an evaluation of the measures characteristics (see IOM, 2010, pp. 69-74).

> **Finding 2-1: The committee finds that partners in the multisectoral health system currently use a vast and complex array of measures of quality in a manner that seems uncoordinated.**

This finding refers to measures of public health relevance, thus excluding measures that are largely pertinent to clinical care. Developing a more coordinated approach would include paying attention to the three purposes of measurement: assessment, improvement, and accountability. A previous IOM committee provided a measurement framework for accountability that acknowledged the different forces at work when accountability is contractually required compared to when accountability is informal or "soft"—what that committee termed "compact accountability" (IOM, 2011a). A challenge identified by the previous committee also persists, in the proliferation of metrics, with limited effort to coordinate, consolidate, and organize in a manner that increases coherence and reduces overlap and duplication.

> **RECOMMENDATION 2-1: The committee recommends that the Department of Health and Human Services and its partners in population health improvement (e.g., public health agencies, health care organizations, and communities) adopt a portfolio of measures of the quality of the multisectoral health system. The portfolio of measures should**
>
> a. **include summary scores reflecting population-level health outcomes and healthy conditions.**
> b. **balance parsimony with sufficient breadth.**
> c. **inform assessment, improvement, and accountability of the multisectoral health system.**

When it refers to summary scores, the committee envisions

- a "healthy outcomes" summary score that is a composite of (the quantitative values for) all outcome measures selected in a portfolio (the summary measures of population health, such as HALE, could serve as such a score, but others could be developed to reflect several different health outcomes of interest); and

- a "healthy conditions" summary score (e.g., such as the community well-being indicator described in IOM [2012]) that is a composite of all intermediate outcomes (or determinants of health) measures selected in a portfolio.

These scores and values could be made publicly available through regular reports and other channels of communication.

A parsimonious (or manageable) portfolio will not be exhaustive or exhausting, it will instead consist of a small number of the most important things, up to, say, four or five per LHI topic. The portfolio will also reflect relevant different areas of the logic model across measures and within each topic, and the measures will not be redundant or overlapping. Measurement has three somewhat overlapping purposes. Measures are needed for the assessment of overall quality in the multisectoral health system, beginning with a focus on governmental public health and health care (where the areas of responsibility and accountability are more clearly delineated) and moving on to the roles and responsibilities of other stakeholders. Measures are also necessary to inform quality improvement and to demonstrate accountability for population health improvement. Measures of quality will inform clinicians and health care organizations, public health agencies, and others in their community health improvement process work at the state and local levels. Measures of quality will also assist members of the public and their elected officials to hold public health officials and other stakeholders, involved in communitywide programs and efforts to improve health, accountable for the quality and effectiveness of their actions (IOM, 2006).

RECOMMENDATION 2-2: The committee recommends that the Department of Health and Human Services and other relevant organizations adopt the following set of criteria for selecting and prioritizing measures of quality for use in population health improvement, including the Leading Health Indicators:

Criteria for conditions or outcomes to be measured
   a. **Reflective of a high preventable burden**[5]
   b. **Actionable at the appropriate level for intervention**

Criteria for the measures
   c. **Timely**
   d. **Usable for assessing various populations**
   e. **Understandable**
   f. **Methodologically rigorous**
   g. **Accepted and harmonized**

Judging the criterion "reflective of a high preventable burden" requires estimates of the frequency of the condition or disease entity and the effectiveness of the interventions. This means that the measures need to refer to interventions and outcomes related to health conditions that account for considerable morbidity and mortality and that are also preventable. A standard measure is needed to determine what is a large burden and what is not, but context matters as well. As an example, the preventable burden of infant mortality is likely relatively small since infant mortality, however catastrophic, is still relatively low. It is likely on the LHI list for several reasons: these are catastrophic events, rates in some groups are much higher than in others, it is an indicator of many issues in the clinical care system and in society as a whole, and it is a measure used in international comparisons. Assessing the evidence of effectiveness may be done by reviewing published findings of the *Guide to Community Preventive Services*, the Cochrane Collaboration, and similar entities. The following characteristics of interventions are important to consider: the feasibility of implementing the intervention (particularly the feasibility in different settings); the potential for improvement (e.g., for a specific health condition, an intervention already delivered at a very high level has less potential for improvement than an equally effective intervention delivered at a lower level); and the extent to which the intervention has externalities (i.e., benefits other conditions or has non-health benefits). The corollary to the "effectiveness of the intervention" condi-

---

[5] The concept of high preventable burden has two components: high burden and existence of effective interventions. This concept (burden × effectiveness), refers to burden as the absolute burden, not relative burden. In other words, a condition like phenylketonuria (PKU) has a high preventable burden if one thinks of the denominator as all people with PKU, but it is a low absolute preventable burden if one uses the entire population.

tion is a case where the magnitude of a problem is such that action is necessary though there is inadequate information on effective interventions (see IOM, 2011a). For example, evidence may be limited to lessons learned or preliminary information on best practices, or there may be multiple potential interacting interventions and insufficient evidence to help pinpoint the most effective. Also, the context of interventions is a critical factor to consider. There are different considerations for measures of relevance to the local level compared to those with relevance to the national level. At the local level, interventions informed by limited evidence, including perhaps emerging best practices or the equivalent, may be tested, so measures of quality are needed. In the absence of evidence-based recommendations from, for example, the *Guide to Community Preventive Services*, interventions or combinations of interventions must have an associated rigorous evaluation.

Although the committee concluded that the nine characteristics of quality in public health do not directly align with measures of quality, it recognizes that a measure that reflects a high preventable burden enables organizations to assess whether their interventions are effective, efficient, equitable (because vulnerable populations may bear a higher burden of, for example, infant mortality) and risk reducing.

The criterion "actionable at the appropriate level of intervention" reflects whether a measure provides sufficient information about a problem to help identify a way to address it, and whether there are effective programs and policies that can be adopted by relevant stakeholders (e.g., local jurisdictions). Finding an effective programs may be done both by referring to systematic reviews, such as those provided by the *Guide to Community Preventive Services* and the Cochrane Collaboration, or by looking to other rigorous efforts to identify best practices, such as the work of the Public Health Law Research program in establishing the Law Atlas, which could in the future help identify associations between changes in policy and health outcomes.[6]

The criterion "timely" refers both to data for a measure (1) being collected frequently enough to make it possible to track changes in the measure that reflect actions intended to affect the outcome or condition and (2) being made available quickly enough (e.g., within 6 months of collection) to be acted on.

"Usable for assessing various populations" means that data are available and can be used to assess different populations (e.g., defined by de-

---

[6] See http://lawatlas.org/about.

mographics or defined by living in a certain zip code) and at different levels (national, state, local).

1. At the total population level and also, to allow levels of equity to be observed, at the subpopulation level (including disparities in every measure).
2. At national, state, and local levels, depending on where policy, programmatic, system, or clinical action is needed. National data include those collected in such systems as the BRFSS, vital records, the American Community Survey, and the Small Area Health Insurance Estimates, while state and local data include those used in the Community Health Status Indicators, drawn from electronic health records, and from other sources used by America's Health Rankings and the County Health Rankings.
3. At levels applicable to the public health system and to the clinical care system where possible.

There are several data-related challenges related to "usable" criterion. There are considerable data limitations at state and local levels and there is a great need for investment in better data infrastructure (an issue that also relates to one of the six drivers of public health quality—metrics and information technology). For example, data needed for all the clinical parameters (e.g., controlled blood pressure, hemoglobin A1c) are unavailable at the local level. Even assuming universal electronic health records (and attaining this was not within reach at the time this report was written), there are many individuals who will remain outside the clinical care system and thus for whom there are no data. For example, uninsured individuals receiving emergency department care may have their blood pressure captured, but without a data generation process similar to that in the National Health and Nutrition Examination Survey, it may not be possible to find out blood pressure levels in a community. Virtually no county has adequate data from BRFSS, and even in the case of large counties, the county-level data are of little value in dealing with the many sub-county issues.

"Understandable" means that no great level of sophistication is required from decision makers, including public health and health care practitioners, policy makers, and the public to understand the criteria. Furthermore, do the measures have face validity? Is the selection process transparent to users and other audiences?

The criterion "methodologically rigorous" refers to the measures having suitable methodological and quantitative characteristics, such as sensitivity, specificity, reliability, validity, and consistency over time and being managed by an established, regularly updated process. The committee believes that a broader criterion is needed because common methodologic criteria such as validity and reliability do not cover issues such as representativeness and consistency. For example, blood pressure control may be a good measure for a clinical care system (i.e., valid and reliable), but a poor measure if the goal is control in the population (which deals with those with poor care, poor adherence, with population-level issues such as physical activity and sodium restriction to reduce population blood pressure levels).

Finally, "accepted and harmonized" refers to measures such as those endorsed by the NQF (primarily focused on health care), or that are in standard use (e.g., used by America's Health Rankings and the County Health Rankings). Difficulties arise, and harmonization is needed, in cases where there are many commonly used measures for the same phenomenon, such as binge drinking and defining an appropriate "norm" in consumption level, or conditions that are not well (or easily) measured, such as major depression in adolescents.

ENDORSING QUALITY MEASURES FOR THE FIELD

In its review of available measures, the committee was unable to find many measures of quality that reside outside the clinical sector. At its information-gathering meeting, the committee learned from participants that the universe of quality measures seems to include very few such measures compared to metrics that aggregate individual-level data related to specific disease states or clinical interventions (Jarris and Stange, 2012).

The report *Priorities for the 2011 National Quality Strategy* (National Priorities Partnership, 2011) contains a table that details priorities, goals, and sample measures organized according to the HHS Three-Part Aim. The section of the table with the heading Population Health is subdivided into three columns: clinical preventive services, healthy lifestyle behaviors, and community health index. The last item refers to truly population health measures (consistent with the Jacobson and Teutsch [2012] definition of "total population health"), and the two sources cited are the County Health Rankings and the AHRQ Prevention Quality Indicators. The former is a portfolio of measures that includes several population-based measures, including health behaviors (e.g., motor vehicle crash death rate and adult obesity), social and economic factors (e.g., high school graduation rates and percentage of children in poverty), and of the physical environment (e.g., drinking water safety and fast food restaurants). The AHRQ Prevention Quality Indicators is a set of individual and composite measures derived from entirely clinical data and designed to assess the effectiveness of a local community's ambulatory health care delivery system.[7] This situation concerning population-based measures suggests that key national efforts to describe health priorities and measures have been predominantly clinical in orientation, as has much of the national effort on quality and prevention, and more attention is warranted for measures related to population-based preventive interventions.

The first step in finding ways to measure quality that are relevant to many different system actors, beginning with public health agencies and health care organizations, could be to find a shared quality language that both health care and public health partners understand (and that can ultimately be understood by stakeholders outside the health sector). For example, the committee began the search for quality measures for the LHIs by reviewing the measures relevant to the LHIs that have been endorsed by the NQF. Where appropriate NQF-endorsed measures do exist, not only are they useful for improving the quality of care, but they can also further progress on the LHIs. This is a linkage that is sometimes not recognized, i.e., that a pediatrician working in a HEDIS-compliant practice setting is not merely working to improve care, but may also be contributing to improving health outcomes at a level far beyond the individual patient.

The advantage offered by having an endorsing entity with an accepted endorsing process is that organizations that want to use measures of quality in their work can simply look to the endorsed sets and select appropriate measures. An endorsement process is one of the first steps in improving measurement and is a prerequisite to the use of standardized measures and measure sets. In order to ensure progress in the formal adoption of population-based measures of quality, an entity charged with endorsing population health measures will need the following characteristics:

- Be nongovernmental, to ensure independence;
- Have the appropriate high-level leadership, organization, and expertise to enable review and endorsement measures of quality intended for population health improvement (e.g., measures of

---

[7] See http://www.qualityindicators.ahrq.gov/Downloads/Modules/PQI/V44/Composite_ User_ Technical_Specification_PQI%20V4.4.pdf (accessed June 26, 2013).

the social and environmental determinants of health), not just measures of clinical care;

- Have processes designed and resourced to evaluate and endorse measures of quality for population health improvement (a process separate and distinct from any existing process for endorsing measures of clinical care); and
- Include expert panel membership and staff support to identify and assess measures of quality for the multisectoral health system, with consideration of data sources, methodology, and other issues that span sectors and disciplines.

Measuring the quality of population-based nonclinical interventions, such as policies, presents more challenges than measuring the quality of individual-based clinical interventions. Clinical interventions can demonstrate improved outcomes in the short term, while population-level action (e.g., clean air laws or universal preschool) may take a generation to bear fruit. For example, evaluating new population health measures will require expertise in interacting with city councils, with planners and land use experts, with educators, and with community organizations. The report *For the Public's Health: The Role of Measurement in Action and Accountability* (IOM, 2011a) asserted that improving population health will require entirely new kinds of measures and data. For example, the authoring committee wrote that

there currently is no coordinated, standard set of true measures of a community's health—not aggregated information about the health of individuals residing in a community, but rather measures of green space, availability of healthy foods, land use and zoning practices that are supportive of health, safety, social capital, and social cohesion, among many other determinants of health. (IOM, 2011a, p. 5)

There currently is no organization that endorses measures of quality to be used for population health (i.e., measures for the multisectoral health system). However, NQF endorses measures of quality for the health care delivery system, and it or a similar entity, appropriately constituted, could perform the same role for the universe of measures that go beyond the health care delivery system.

Given the conclusions of IOM committees and other groups that health care is only responsible for a modest proportion of the factors that influence population health, the committee calls for changes in the approach to measurement of quality.

RECOMMENDATION 2-3: The committee recommends that the Department of Health and Human Services ensure the implementation of a systematic approach to develop and manage a portfolio of measures of quality for the multisectoral health system. HHS also should establish or designate a nongovernmental and appropriately equipped entity to endorse measures of quality.

An entity endorsing measures of quality for the multisectoral health system would need to be guided by a strong research infrastructure, elements of which were described in a recommendation in an earlier report (IOM, 2012) that called for a research agenda and funding to support the public health research and evaluation infrastructure. Also, an endorsing entity would not have to be, and ideally will not be, an organization that develops measures; although the two skillsets overlap somewhat, the roles and purposes are very different. With regard to the role of HHS in systematizing the approach to measures of quality, the committee has learned about two evolving HHS activities in the area of quality measurement. These are the Centers for Medicare & Medicaid Services (CMS) Quality Measures Task Force and the HHS Interagency Measurement Policy Council. The CMS Task Force is charged with "developing recommendations on CMS measure implementation with the goal of aligning and prioritizing measures across programs and avoidance of duplication or conflict among developing and implemented measures" and one of its goals is to coordinate "measure implementation, development and measurement policies" with other agencies in HHS (Goodrich, 2012). The Measurement Policy Council, which was established in 2012 as a subgroup of the HHS National Quality Strategy effort, is focused on policies for measure development, implementation, and alignment across HHS. The council includes AHRQ, CMS, the Office of the National Coordinator for Health Information Technology, the Substance Abuse and Mental Health Services Administration, the HHS Office of the Assistant Secretary for Planning and Evaluation, the Health Resources and Services Administration, CDC, the Office of Minority Health, the Food and Drug Administration, and others. Its initial focus is on "alignment and prioritization of measures in six major areas: hypertension, smoking cessation, depression, health care acquired conditions, patient experience, and care coordination" (Goodrich, 2012). It appears that the HHS-wide council, like the CMS Task Force, is largely oriented toward clinical care. Moreover, if the objective is to improve the health of the population by creating healthy conditions, coordination and measures are needed that involve sectors of government beyond HHS, for example, the array of executive branch leaders (including the Departments of Education, Housing, and Transportation) participating in the National Prevention, Health Promotion, and Public Health Council.

Data and information are needed to identify and develop measures of quality, and to support the development and management of the portfolio of measures described in Recommendation 2-3. Strengthening public health agency capacity in this area will also spur progress in the priority area for quality improvement in public health "Metrics and Information Technology." To this end, the committee endorses both Recommendations 1 and 2 from the 2011 IOM report *For the Public's Health: The Role of Measurement in Action and Accountability*, and Recommendation 6 from the 2012 IOM report *For the Public's Health: Investing in a Healthier Future*. The former called for strengthening the population health information infrastructure, and for integrating, aligning, and standardizing health data and health outcome measurement at all geographic levels.[8] The latter called for a research infrastructure to establish the value of public health and prevention strategies, mechanisms for their effective implementation, health and economic outcomes derived, and the comparative effectiveness and impact of those strategies.[9]

---

[8] Recommendation 1: The committee recommends that: (1) The Secretary of Health and Human Services transform the mission of the National Center for Health Statistics to provide leadership to a renewed population health information system through enhanced coordination, new capacities, and better integration of the determinants of health. (2) The National Prevention, Health Promotion, and Public Health Council include in its annual report to Congress on its national prevention and health-promotion strategy an update on the progress of the National Center for Health Statistics transformation.

Recommendation 2: The committee recommends that the Department of Health and Human Services support and implement the following to integrate, align, and standardize health data and health-outcome measurement at all geographic levels:

     a.   A core, standardized set of indicators that can be used to assess the health of communities.

     b.   A core, standardized set of health-outcome indicators for national, state, and local use.

     c.   A summary measure of population health that can be used to estimate and track health-adjusted life expectancy for the United States.

[9] Recommendation 6: The committee recommends that Congress direct the Department of Health and Human Services to develop a robust research infrastructure for establishing the effectiveness and value of public health and prevention strategies, mechanisms for effective implementation of these strategies, the health and economic outcomes derived from this investment, and the comparative effectiveness and impact of this investment. The infrastructure should include

- A dedicated stream of funding for research and evaluation.
- A national research agenda.

RECOMMENDATION 2-4: The Department of Health and Human Services should develop, implement, and support data collection, analysis, and dissemination mechanisms and infrastructure for the portfolio of quality measures so they are usable for health assessment and improvement at the national, state, and local levels.

The committee hopes that the implementation of all IOM recommendations in this area will contribute to future data systems that address current limitations. The ability to develop good quality measures requires ensuring that timely data are available at national, state and, in particular, local levels, and that these data can be stratified for vulnerable sub-populations to assess changes in health disparities during improvement efforts.

- Development of data systems and measures to capture research-quality information on key elements of public health delivery, including program implementation costs.
- Development and validation of methods for comparing the benefits and costs of alternative strategies to improve population health.

3

Measures of Quality

The committee was charged with identifying measures of quality for the Leading Health Indicators (LHIs), and in this chapter it provides a starter set of measures identified by developing detailed versions of the logic models introduced in Chapter 1 for four of the LHI topic areas: tobacco; environmental quality (the air quality LHI); obesity, nutrition, and physical activity; and maternal, infant, and child health.

As noted earlier, the committee believes that the purpose of measurement is threefold. Assessment can be conducted simply for the purpose of monitoring and reporting about the health of a population; this can be done to provide a comparison with other jurisdictions or nations, or to mobilize interested parties. Measures can be used in the work of quality improvement, whether organization-wide or in a specific program. And measures can be used for accountability, for example, to report back to funders, partners, legislators, and communities. More extensive discussion of the three purposes of measurement is provided in the Institute of Medicine (IOM) report *For the Public's Health: The Role of Measurement in Action and Accountability* (2011a, p. 3, et seq.).

In addition to the criteria outlined in Chapter 2, several other issues are important when selecting measures of quality. The level of measurement is important, for example. Some of the LHIs are national in scope and dependent on national-level data, but they may be of secondary importance in some local jurisdictions. One of the challenges in measurement is the paucity of truly granular health data at the local level and the capability to access and analyze the data that are available. A variety of novel strategies for data collection and analysis are needed to expand the data sources available to local public health planners and their system partners. Data relevant to health are also available from non-health sources, such as police records and school data, as well as other nontraditional sources such as Google Maps for parks and Chamber of Commerce and trade groups for businesses and tax revenues. As one example of evolution in analytical capabilities, Srebotnjak and colleagues (2010) developed a novel methodology to estimate health trends (e.g., diagnosed diabetes) in counties and other small population areas. Their modeling approach allows health officials and researchers to use Behavioral Risk Factor Surveillance System (BRFSS) data for small-area estimation and validation. Advances in information and communication technology offer novel opportunities for data generation, such as crowdsourcing data collection and analysis to support health improvement (e.g., through health behavior change) in the community (see, for example, Piniewski et al., 2011). A real-life application is offered by the experience with Global Positioning System (GPS)-equipped inhalers (i.e., the Asthmapolis sensor and mobile application system that produces "timely, comprehensive and objective data on the burden of asthma"[1] but also supports remote monitoring of broncho-dilator use; see Van Sickle et al. [2013]). There are several challenges in creating novel data sources, including balancing business potential with public use, and addressing concerns about real and perceived threats to privacy, technical obstacles related to gleaning useful information from "big" data, and the cost of establishing and sustaining long-term data generation and analysis efforts. However, the potential of disruptive innovation to dramatically increase access to population health data is undeniable.

The committee did not conduct a systematic and comprehensive review of all potential measures related to the LHIs for several reasons. Such an undertaking would require time and resources (including a wider range of expertise) to research all effective interventions for a given outcome, and to identify and evaluate all candidate measures. The committee also believes that describing a framework and process for a continually updated set of measures could be of more lasting value than identifying a static set of measures. Finally, many measures of quality relate to the specific interventions implemented and are context specific. For this reason, too, describing a process seemed more useful than providing specific examples that would result from applying that process.

As discussed earlier, the LHIs are heterogeneous, and organizing them to support quality improvement is not a straightforward process. There are at least three ways to conceptually organize the *Healthy People 2020* LHIs other than the alphabetical order presented in the Healthy People publications. They may be organized roughly according to the

---

[1] Available at http://asthmapolis.com/public-health (accessed June 26, 2013).

ecological model,[2] based on the type of "determinant" of health/level in the ecological model they occupy. They may be divided by locus of intervention (clinical/individual vs. population-based), al-though some LHIs fall somewhere in between. LHIs do not fit neatly into one level of the ecological model, and may be altered by interventions at both the individual and at the population level. Finally, the LHIs may be organized according to the committee's logic model provided above: resources and capacity, interventions, healthy conditions, and healthy outcomes, with a focus on the latter two categories, which can "house" most of the LHIs (see Figure 3-1).

Table 3-1 provides a list of the LHIs organized according to the logic model (and shown in bold type), and showing areas for potential measures of quality related to the LHIs. The non-bolded entries represent non-LHI measures that are directly linked to an LHI (e.g., an intermediate outcome linked to the LHIs representing an ultimate health outcome) or found along the pathway that includes an LHI (e.g., morbidity from childhood disease is an ultimate outcome linked to the LHI childhood vaccines). The entries marked with an asterisk represent measures that are endorsed by the National Quality Forum (NQF), that met the criteria for inclusion in the County Health Rankings, or that met other criteria such as face validity in the case of measures that emerge from the evidence-based interventions recommended by the *Guide to Community Preventive Services* (population-based interventions) and the U.S. Preventive Services Task Force (USPSTF) (for interventions in the clinical

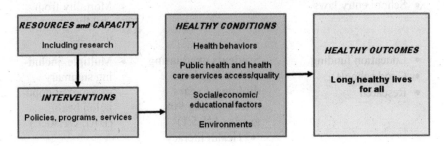

FIGURE 3-1 Health outcome logic model.

---

[2] The ecological model is a diagram adapted from Dahlgren and Whitehead (1991) by an IOM committee and in *Healthy People 2020* planning by the Department of Health and Human Services (HHS) to show the array of determinants of health, or the ecology of health, beginning with individual level factors at the center (biology/genetics), then on to behavior, family, social networks, and communities, followed by broad policies pertaining to the determinants of health (education, income, etc.) at the state and national level (see HHS, 2008; IOM, 2003a).

setting). The table is not intended to be comprehensive or exhaustive, but the committee hopes that it illustrates a step in the process of identifying measures of quality related to the LHI. A subsequent step would be the application of the criteria outlined in Chapter 2.

TABLE 3-1 The LHIs (in Bold Typeface) Organized According to the Logic Model and Showing Areas for and Examples of Potential Measures of Quality (in Regular Typeface)

Resources and Capacity; Interventions	Healthy Conditions	Outcome
• Title X, Medicaid family planning waivers • Family planning services	**Females receiving reproductive health services (FP-7.1)** • Teen birth rate* • Children using age-appropriate restraints in motor vehicles • Children in poverty*	**Infant deaths (MICH-1.3)** **Preterm births (MICH-9.1)** • Low birth weight*
• Funding for vaccine and services for un- or under-insured • School entry laws	**Childhood vaccines (IID-8)**	• Morbidity from childhood diseases • Mortality from childhood diseases
• Education funding • Good schools • Research	**Students graduating with a regular diploma 4 years after starting 9th grade (AH-5.1)***[a] • Health literacy • Unemployment rate	• Multiple, including summary measure of population health (HALY/HALE)

TABLE 3-1 Continued

Resources and Capacity; Interventions	Healthy Conditions	Outcome
• Funding for HIV screening services • Communication and education efforts	**Persons living with HIV who know their serostatus (HIV-13)**	• HIV incidence • HIV mortality
• Increasing alcohol taxes; enhanced enforcement of laws prohibiting sales to minors* • Research	**Adolescents (12-17 years old) using alcohol or any illicit drugs (SA-13.1)** **Adults engaging in binge drinking (SA-14.3)**	**Fatal injuries (IVP-1.1)**
• Incentives to use public transportation, CAFE standards • Research (on ways to reduce children's ETS exposure) • State and local smoke-free policies • Excise taxes • Increased unit price on tobacco products*[b]	**Air Quality Index (EH-1)** Daily particulate matter days (PM$_{2.5}$)* **Children exposed to secondhand smoke (TU-11.1)** **Adolescents who smoke (TU-2.2)** **Adults who smoke (TU-1.1)***	• Cardiovascular and respiratory mortality[c] • (also **Infant deaths**)
• Passage and enforcement of mental health parity laws • Coverage of mental health services	• Access to mental health services. • Youth access to unsecured firearms*[d]	**Suicides (MHMD-1)** **Adolescents experiencing major depressive episodes (MHMD-4.1)**

TABLE 3-1 Continued

Resources and Capacity; Interventions	Healthy Conditions	Outcome
• Effective law enforcement • Use of evidence-based substance use prevention services in schools and communities • State policies regarding firearms[e]	• Schools implementing school-based interventions aimed at reducing youth violence*	Homicides (IVP-29)
• Ratio of population to dentists* • Increased reimbursement levels for adult and child oral health services under Medicaid **Persons with a usual primary care provider (AHS-3)** **Persons with medical insurance (AHS-1.1)** • Percent of population under age 65 without health insurance* • The Affordable Care Act	**Persons using the oral health care system (OH-7)** • Preventable hospitalization	• HALY/HALE • OH3.1, OH3.2, OH3.3, OH1.1[f]
• Local public health monitoring of hypertension rates and support to provider community	**Adults with hypertension under control (HDS-12)**	• HALY/HALE • Cardiovascular and stroke mortality

TABLE 3-1 Continued

Resources and Capacity; Interventions	Healthy Conditions	Outcome
• Local health plan and purchaser monitoring of colorectal cancer screening rates • Reimbursement of preventive services	**Adults receiving colorectal cancer screening (C-16)**	• Colorectal cancer mortality
• Access to recreational facilities* • Diabetic screening* • Proportion of clinicians screening for obesity at age 6 and older and offering or referring to comprehensive, intensive behavioral interventions[g] • Behavioral interventions to reduce screen time (*Community Guide*) • Increased physical activity in school • "Urban design and land use policies and practices that support physical activity in small geographic areas (generally a few blocks)"*[h]	**Adults meeting physical activity guidelines (PA-2.4)** **Total vegetable intake (NWS-15.1)** **Adult diabetic population with poor glucose control (D-5.1)** **Adults who are obese (NWS-9)** **Children and adolescents who are obese (NWS-10.4)** • Limited access to healthy foods* • Fast food restaurants*	• HALY/HALE

NOTE: Items marked with an asterisk (*) represent measures that are endorsed by NQF, met the criteria for inclusion in the County Health Rankings, or met other criteria (e.g., face validity in the case of measures that emerge from the evidence-based interventions recommended by the *Guide to Community Preventive Services* [population-based interventions] and the U.S. Preventive Services Task Force [for interventions in the clinical setting]).

[a] "The averaged freshman graduation rate measures the percentage of public high school students who graduate on time with a regular diploma" (Department of Education, National Center for Education Statistics, 2012, http://nces.ed.gov/programs/coe/analysis/2012-section5.asp [accessed June 1, 2013]).

TABLE 3-1 Continued

---

[b] Tworek et al., 2010.

[c] See Henschel et al., 2012, for a review of published studies of air pollution interventions which showed that improving air quality is associated with improved health outcomes (decreased respiratory and cardiovascular morbidity and mortality).

[d] Baxley and Miller, 2006.

[e] Fleegler et al., 2013, found that "a higher number of firearm laws in a state was associated with a lower rate of firearm fatalities in the state" controlling for a range of factors, but also concluded that additional research is needed to examine the nature of the association.

[f] OH-1.1: Reduce (by 10%, from 33.3% to 30.0%) the proportion of young children aged 3 to 5 years with dental caries experience in their primary teeth; OH-3.1: Reduce (by 10%, from 27.8% to 25%) the proportion of adults aged 35 to 44 years with untreated dental decay; OH-3.2: Reduce (by 10%, from 17.1% to 15.4%) the proportion of older adults aged 65 to 74 years with untreated coronal caries; and OH-3.3: Reduce (by 10%, from 37.9% to 34.1%) the proportion of older adults aged 75 years and older with untreated root surface caries.

[g] "The DGAs (2005 *Dietary Guidelines for Americans*) provide science based guidelines for food policy, food benefits, and nutrition education provided through the Federal nutrition assistance programs. The 2005 DGA Advisory Committee Report stated that 'greater consumption of fruits and vegetables (5-13 servings or 2½-6½ cups per day depending on calorie needs) is associated with a reduced risk of stroke and perhaps other cardiovascular diseases, with a reduced risk of cancers in certain sites (oral cavity and pharynx, larynx, lung, esophagus, stomach, and colon-rectum), and with a reduced risk of type 2 diabetes (vegetables more than fruit). Moreover, increased consumption of fruits and vegetables may be a useful component of programs designed to achieve and sustain weight loss'" (USDA, 2008).

[h] *Guide to Community Preventive Services*, 2004.

The committee considered the quality improvement needs at all geographic levels, with the recognition that as one localizes quality improvement it becomes more important to have measures most relevant to the interventions chosen (which are intrinsically more process-oriented or structurally oriented) and which are more likely to be measurable and changeable at local levels. To reconcile these somewhat different objectives, the committee suggests that a well-developed portfolio of measures will have a core set of standard measures to be used at all levels (national, state, local), and a menu of additional options (largely process measures appropriate to specific settings) to be used as needed at the local level.

The priority areas or drivers of improvement of quality in public health identified in the work of the OASH (Honoré and Scott, 2010) are metrics and information technology; evidence-based practices, research, and evaluation; systems thinking; sustainability and stewardship; policy;

and workforce and education. As with the quality characteristics, these drivers cannot be linked directly to LHIs, but instead refer to the system's underlying structural inputs illustrated by the Resources and Capacity box in Figure 3-1. For public health agencies, these may be linked with domains and measures employed in the Public Health Accreditation Board voluntary accreditation process. The drivers also seem somewhat related to the notion of foundational capabilities (part of a minimum package of public health services) proposed by a recent IOM report (2012). Those capabilities include the research infrastructure, information systems, and skills and workforce development for policy analysis and communication. That committee recommended that the minimum package, including the foundational capabilities, be used to establish new and robust approaches to demonstrating accountability, including linking funding inputs to outcomes in order to demonstrate value to funders and the public.

Below, the committee provides a "starter set" of measures of quality that could be considered in the development of a robust portfolio of measures for the nation, and for state and local jurisdictions. The committee used two approaches.

1. The committee found that many of the LHIs included or led to one or more measures that can be used to measure quality (see Table 3-1).
2. The committee developed case studies that applied the report's health outcome logic model to the LHI topic areas of
   a. tobacco use;
   b. nutrition, physical activity, and obesity;
   c. environmental quality; and
   d. maternal, infant, and child health.

Finding 3-1: The committee finds that

    a. **Many of the Leading Health Indicators are measures of health outcomes or of conditions that can directly affect health outcomes and are, therefore, measures of the quality of the multisectoral health system.**

    b. **The LHIs that meet the definition above of a quality measure can be used for assessment, improvement, and accountability. To be used thus, they must be relevant and measurable at the national, state, and local levels.**

    c. The LHIs reflect conditions or outcomes that direct-
ly contribute to the *Healthy People 2020* foundation
measures (e.g., general health status, health-related
quality of life) and the ecologic model that underlies it.

FOUR CASE STUDIES

The committee has developed concrete illustrations of the functioning of the logic model for four LHI topics and also more detailed expla-
nation of activities for each LHI topic to help in the selection of metrics.
Each case study lists the LHIs under the topic, provides a brief digest of
the evidence and causal pathway(s) to which the LHI is an endpoint (ultimate outcome) or an intermediate outcome, provides a detailed logic
model to illustrate the possible measures under Healthy Conditions and
Health Outcomes, depicts the likely relationships among them, and offers
both a list of possible measures and a shorter list of candidate measures
(endorsed by NQF; based on evidence from the *Guide to Community
Preventive Services*, the USPSTF, or equivalent, and for which data
sources are available). The 1997 IOM report *Improving Health in the
Community: A Role for Performance Monitoring* provides additional lists
of potential measures organized by topic.

The detailed examples and their associated logic models provide an
overview of resources, interventions, conditions, and outcomes that are
related to specific and important health determinants and outcomes, and
highlight the importance of the LHIs as components of these models. By
explicitly describing these relationships, these models provide ideas for
potential measures for assessing (1) the effectiveness of resources, programs, and actions on conditions that promote health, and (2) the impact
of these conditions on outcomes. As the committee's Recommendation
1-1 states, these conditions and outcomes are a reflection of the quality
of the multisectoral health system. Similar models can be developed for
other health determinants (or healthy conditions) and outcomes related to
other Leading Health Indicators, or to other Healthy People objectives.
These models can also facilitate the development of more detailed and
quantitative systems models, such as Prevention Impacts Simulation
Model (PRISM) and Population Health Model (POHEM), described earlier in this report, that can identify which components of these models
make greater potential contributions to improved health conditions and
outcomes. As mentioned above, evidence from studies and meta-
analyses, such as those of the *Guide to Clinical Preventive Services* and
Guide to Community Preventive Services, and practical knowledge sup-

port some of the logical relationships and connections in these models, but evidence to support—or refute—other relationships is sorely needed. Thus, another use of these models is to highlight relationships supported by scientific evidence that can already serve as the foundation for measures of health system quality, while also identifying other relationships in need of further study.

By way of illustration, the committee used the tobacco model to identify potential measures of quality. Outcome-related quality measures can be generated from "tobacco-related disease, functional losses, and mortality." Obvious examples include lung cancer incidence and mortality, and the prevalence of and mortality from chronic obstructive pulmonary disease, to which tobacco use is a major contributor. There are several potential healthy condition-related quality measures that are suggested by the model. "Prevalence of tobacco use" is most closely related to outcomes and is the most obvious choice for a quality measure. The seven conditions shown that directly affect "prevalence of tobacco use" could next be reviewed for those which have the greatest potential impact, the best supporting scientific evidence for their effectiveness, and available data to track them (see Recommendation 2-2). Depending on need, one or more of these seven conditions could be selected to monitor performance of the health system. Most of the process measures in the model are supported by evidence and recommended by either the *Clinical Guide* or the *Community Guide*. Again, these require review using the selection criteria described in Recommendation 2-2. Because these actions and processes can be implemented at the state and local level, selecting one or more of them as the basis for a measure of state or local health system performance could provide more immediate feedback to local public health practitioners and stakeholders than relying on quality measures of conditions and outcomes, which change over a much longer time frame.

The case studies gave the committee an opportunity to consider the nine characteristics of public health quality and the six drivers of public health quality improvement as they relate primarily to the Resources and Capacity component of the logic model. As discussed in Chapter 1, in general, the nine characteristics cannot be directly linked with quality measures, since they primarily describe the system itself (e.g., population-centered, transparent, health-promoting) and the interventions undertaken to address health issues (a program or process or policy may be risk-reducing, or may be a manifestation of the system's vigilance, or efficiency). Below, the committee provides tobacco use as an example for applying the nine characteristics of quality and the six drivers. Additionally, decision makers can maintain a focus on quality by asking themselves if an intervention being considered is consistent with the nine characteristics, or if it reveals something about the system that resonates with the nine characteristics. For example, in the case of the tobacco LHI, one would expect interventions in use or under consideration to be congruent with one of more of the following:

- **effective:** based on evidence about what works to decrease tobacco use and its initiation, and showing system (or an agency's) capacity to identify and implement effective interventions;
- **efficient:** cost-effective, providing value on investment, demonstrating the capacity to invest wisely;
- **equitable:** reaching the appropriate target population, paying attention to vulnerable populations;
- **health-promoting:** ensuring that interventions to decrease tobacco use increase the probability of healthy conditions (including healthy behaviors) and outcomes;
- **population-centered:** intended to protect and promote health and healthy (e.g., smoke-free) environments for everyone;
- **proactive:** timely and responsive to emerging data and issues, and even able to predict and prepare (e.g., for legislative or regulatory challenges);
- **risk-reducing:** having identified areas of risk, this would reflect on the capacity of those implementing interventions to mitigate the probability of negative outcomes or protect against risk;
- **transparent:** for example, engaging the community, communicate openly about objectives and strategies, and make data and information widely available; and
- **vigilant:** include such activities as surveillance and simulation modeling to inform about what works and to what extent it is working.

The drivers of quality (population health metrics and information technology; evidence-based practices, research, and evaluation; systems thinking; sustainability and stewardship; policy; and public health workforce and education) are consistent with the foundational capabilities of public health described in the 2012 IOM report *For the Public's Health: Investing in a Healthier Future*. These drivers refer to system elements that are needed for all topics and hence they are described here rather than for each case study to reduce redundancy. For example, systems thinking, policy, and workforce considerations apply to most health improvement efforts, whether in tobacco use reduction or in decreasing preterm births. Below, the committee discusses how the six drivers provide a clear starting point for improving quality in public health in the area of tobacco use. Specifically, health departments (and some of their partners in communities) will need

1. The data and information technology capabilities to understand the extent and nature of tobacco use in their communities. This could be achieved independently, for large and better-resourced health departments, or through various collaborative arrangements for smaller health departments. This is also essential for information exchange with health care providers in the community. Gathering data about providers who implement the National Committee for Quality Assurance (NCQA) measure of asking about tobacco use at every patient encounter and providing counseling when needed could contribute considerably to improving tobacco use behaviors in their community and to public health officials' understanding of how comprehensively an effective intervention is being delivered.

2. The ability to conduct or access research and evaluation in order to enable evidence-based practice in tobacco use prevention and reduction. Quality measures in this area could be informed by building on an already robust evidence base.

3. Systems thinking that recognizes the complex and reinforcing network of causes and effects that influences tobacco use. Factors contributing to smoking and other tobacco use behavior include social norms; the existence of adequate laws and policies and their enforcement, the availability of counseling and other smoking-cessation supports, health insurance coverage of smoking-cessation services including access to pharmacologic products (nicotine replacement therapy and others); and multiple actors who can influence tobacco use, such as the mass media, employers, local governments, and schools. Smoking, in turn, is a factor in the causal trajectories of cardiovascular disease, many cancers, respiratory diseases, and other health outcomes. Similarly to other LHIs, tobacco use is a health issue that involves many areas of society, including government, schools, workplaces, community organizations, and the mass and entertainment media. The ability to mobilize and sustain effective multisector

      partnerships requires a skillset considerably linked with systems thinking.

4. Sustainability and stewardship that have relevance to how interventions are crafted, for example, dedicating tobacco tax revenues to tobacco use prevention (rather than going to general revenues) and requiring the inclusion of nicotine replacement therapy in insurance coverage. Stewardship also offers an opportunity to talk about the health system and mutual accountability of diverse contributors for changes that improve health (see IOM, 2011a).

5. Policy-development capabilities, including legal counsel and other expert staff who can advise local or state government about changes in policies, regulations, and laws to extend and sustain public health successes; this includes doing the research and health impact assessments, developing the legal framework, getting community support, engaging in advocacy, etc.

6. Workforce and education, in particular, the need for public health department and community organization staff who are trained in policy analysis and development and in communication (including social marketing, the use of social media, etc.).

Resources and capabilities analogous to those described above are needed for improvement efforts related to most of the LHI topics.

Tobacco

      There are two Leading Health Indicators under the LHI topic Tobacco Use: adults who are current cigarette smokers (TU-1.1) and adolescents who smoked cigarettes in the past 30 days (TU-2.2). (The Environmental Quality topic includes the related LHI "Children aged 3 to 11 years exposed to secondhand smoke" [TU-11.1].)

      The committee applied the Health Outcome Logic Model to the topic of Tobacco Use. This included reviewing the evidence base on effective interventions, such as clinical services, programs, laws, and policies among other system inputs, the healthy conditions needed to decrease poor tobacco use–related outcomes, and finally, the intermediate and ultimate outcomes of decreased tobacco use. The committee identified a set of quality measures, and also explained how consideration of the six drivers of improvement of quality in public health would influence action to reduce tobacco use.

First, the committee reviewed how tobacco interventions and programs relate to health outcomes. A scan of the literature showed a strong evidence base for interventions that reduce or prevent the initiation of tobacco use. Recommendations on effective tobacco control interventions have been provided by the USPSTF, the *Guide to Community Preventive Services*, the Cochrane Collaboration, and others. *Ending the Tobacco Epidemic*, a 2010 HHS strategic plan, reviewed three additional authoritative sources on tobacco control programs (HHS, 2010). The common findings across all these sources are that the most effective programs are comprehensive, sustained, and accountable, and the HHS plan found that five specific types of interventions collectively reduce tobacco use: mass-media counter-marketing campaigns targeting youth; the adoption of comprehensive smoke-free laws; the availability of affordable tobacco-cessation options; excise tax increases that raise the retail price of tobacco products; and restrictions on advertising and promotion (HHS, 2010). Research has also shown that even when a population-level intervention has only modest effects on tobacco use behavior, the public health impact can be large (National Cancer Institute, 2000).

Second, the committee reviewed the literature on some of the inputs, such as system resources and capacity, programs, and policies. Examples include evidence that taxes and other policies are effective and may even bring in revenue and evidence that greater spending by states on specific types of tobacco interventions leads to the desired health outcomes, which are reductions in tobacco use, reductions in health conditions that result from tobacco use, and ultimately, increased healthy life expectancy. Research has shown that states and localities that have made substantial investments in comprehensive tobacco control programs have realized faster decreases in cigarette sales and smoking prevalence (HHS, 2010).

In its search for quality measures that could be used for the Tobacco Use LHIs, the committee found that NQF has endorsed a set of tobacco use measures. Most are for use in the clinical setting, and only two seem suited to the level of the total population: children who are exposed to secondhand smoke inside the home (a measure from the Maternal and Child Health Bureau of the Health Resources and Services Administration [HRSA]) and adult smoking prevalence (a measure from the Centers for Disease Control and Prevention [CDC]). However, there are no endorsed measures of population or community-level factors that influence tobacco use, such as the prevalence of smoke-free laws in a state or community (such as laws that ban smoking in multi-unit rental housing, a factor that could play a role in child exposure to environmental tobacco smoke).

Making the best use of evidence about the effectiveness of many policy-based interventions to prevent and reduce tobacco use by both adolescents and adults requires a certain level of capacity within health departments, which are, according to the IOM Committee on Public Health Strategies to Improve Health, "a source of knowledge and analysis on community and population health" (the assessment and policy development functions of public health) and "a steward of the community's health, assuring that policies and services needed for a healthy population are in place" (the policy development and assurance functions of public health) (IOM, 2012). Each community, state, or measure-endorsing entity could use the logic model described below to generate a portfolio of measures for comparison and improvement in the area of tobacco use. The logic model (see Figure 3-2, page 62) can also be used to assess local resources and capacities to implement interventions to reduce or prevent tobacco use.

Tobacco Use: Example Measures of Quality

Measures of Healthy Outcomes (Outcome Measures)

   Lung cancer mortality
   Prevalence of chronic obstructive pulmonary disease

Measures of Healthy Conditions (Intermediate Outcome Measures)

   Percentage of adults who smoke
   Unit price of tobacco products
   Availability of tobacco products
   Availability of smoking cessation programs
   Insurance coverage for nicotine replacement therapy
   Availability of policies regulating tobacco use in multi-unit housing
   Percentage of active smokers trying to quit (Farkas et al., 1996)
   Percentage of workplaces covered by smoke-free workplace policies

Measures of Interventions (Process) or Resources (Structure)

   Comprehensive smoke-free laws

Mass-media counter marketing campaigns, especially targeting youth
Excise tax on tobacco products
Accessible, affordable, and effective tobacco cessation programs

The following measures are endorsed by NQF (measure steward provided in parentheses):

- Medical assistance with smoking and tobacco use cessation (NCQA)
- Screening and cessation interventions (American Medical Association [AMA] Convened Consortium for Performance Improvement)
- Adult current smoking prevalence (CDC)
- Risky behavior assessment or counseling by age 13 years (NCQA)
- Screening for abdominal aortic aneurysm in adult male smokers (ActiveHealth Management)

Nutrition, Physical Activity, and Obesity

There are four LHIs under the LHI topic Nutrition, Physical Activity, and Obesity: adults who meet guidelines on physical activity (aerobic and muscle strengthening), obese adults, obese children, and adequate vegetable intake in persons 2 years of age and older. These are process measures along the trajectory to the outcomes of premature mortality, such as from cardiovascular disease, complications of diabetes, and cancer.

The evidence base in these related areas is growing rapidly, but it is not as robust as the evidence on interventions to reduce tobacco use; considerable gaps remain. Thus, the obesity model (and others) provided can be used to select potential quality measures, but it can also be used to identify components and relationships needing additional research. For example, several actions and processes depicted in the obesity model have face validity as potential quality measures, but lack scientific evidence about their effectiveness because of limited research. Even some of the conditions depicted in the model as contributing to "reduced prevalence of obesity" lack adequate scientific evidence about their effectiveness. The obesity example and model, therefore, provide fewer potential quality measures, particularly for processes and conditions, and

62

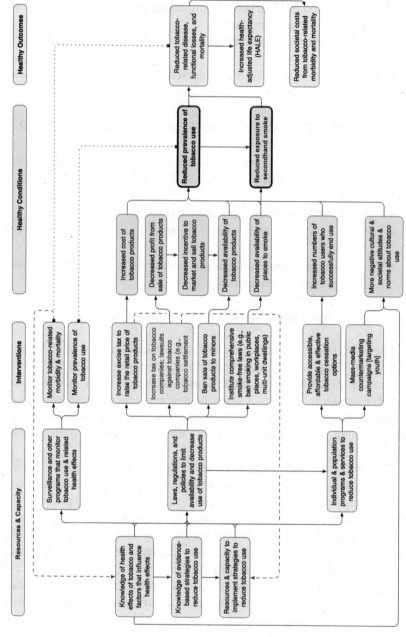

FIGURE 3-2 Applying the logic model to the LHI topic Tobacco Use.

highlight the need for additional research. At this time, quality measures for this topic area might be limited to "prevalence of obesity," for which there is good evidence about its impact on specific diseases and functional status, and outcomes with a direct link to obesity, such as diabetes, cardiovascular disease, and mobility.

Obesity is an area where multiple determinants of health are involved, and the causal pathways are extremely complex. In addition to individual level factors, such as genetics, there are behavioral factors that include nutrition and physical activity (and two of the LHIs measure these), and a wide range of factors in the built and social environment. The built and social environment factors include the availability and affordability of healthy foods, especially fruit and vegetables, in the community and in schools; the availability and quality of a public transportation system (associated with increased walking); and the quality of the built environment, including the density of fast food outlets, the availability of green spaces such as parks and walking or bike trails, and the existence of complete streets that allow safe access to pedestrians of varying physical ability and to bicycles (i.e., those with sidewalks, bike lanes, wheelchair ramps, and signals appropriate for people with vision impairments) (Gustat et al., 2012; McCormack and Shiell, 2011; Saelens and Handy, 2008). Socioeconomic status and race/ethnicity are linked in complex ways to the environmental characteristics just described, for instance, families and communities that live in or near poverty are more likely to live in environments that are less health-promoting. Social norms also play an important role in shaping public perception of eating and physical activity behaviors and environments, as they have in the case of tobacco use. Some process measures related to the LHI obesity have been identified, but additional research is needed to develop and validate relevant process measures or measures of intermediate outcomes and health conditions, such as walkability indices (Christian et al., 2011). Research on aspects of the built environment and the information environment (e.g., advertising) is ongoing. It will be important to establish whether menu labeling policies have an effect on consumer behavior and some early affirmative evidence is emerging (Krieger et al., 2013).

The logic model described below (see Figure 3-3, page 65) could be used by organizations identifying measures of quality (or a measure-endorsing entity) in the area of nutrition, physical activity, and obesity. The logic model can also be used to assess local resources and capacities to implement interventions to improve nutritional status and physical activity, and to reduce obesity.

Nutrition, Physical Activity, and Obesity:
Example Measures of Quality

Measures of Outcome

Mortality rate from disease with obesity as a risk factor
Percent of overweight and obese adults
Percent of overweight and obese children
Expected quality of life in the population
Number of disability days due to obesity related disease
Number of quality nutrition programs available

Measures of Healthy Conditions (e.g., Intermediate Outcomes)

Number of adults with regular physical activity
Number of child hours watching television (or hours of screen time)
Number of adults following nutritional guidelines
Amount of calorie intake in diets
Number of hours children are active during school days
Number of months children were breastfed

Measures of Resources (Structure) or Interventions (Process)

Number of programs that promote physical activity for children
Availability of fresh fruits and produce
Nutritious meals available in school, day care, and assisted-living housing
Space available for physical activity in child care and school facilities
Menu labeling regulations
Average calories per meal purchased at chain restaurants

The following measures have been endorsed by NQF (measure steward provided in parentheses):

- Child overweight or obesity status based on parental report of body mass index (Maternal and Child Health Bureau, HRSA)
- Weight assessment and counseling for nutrition and physical activity for children and adolescents (NCQA)

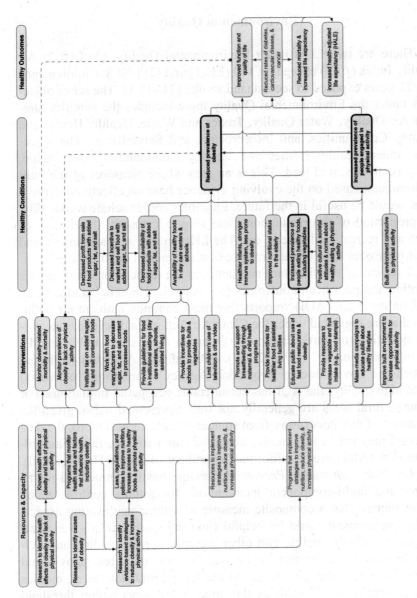

FIGURE 3-3 Applying the logic model to the LHI topic Nutrition, Physical Activity, and Obesity.

Environmental Quality

There are two LHIs under Environmental Quality: (1) LHI 7: Air Quality Index (AQI) exceeding 100 (EH-1) and (2) LHI 8: Children aged 3 to 11 years exposed to secondhand smoke (TU-11.1). The set of objectives under the Environmental Quality topic includes the subtitles Outdoor Air Quality, Water Quality, Toxics and Waste, Healthy Homes and Healthy Communities, and Infrastructure and Surveillance. The objectives under Healthy Homes and Healthy Communities cover radon, mold, pesticides, and lead. This is an area where measures of the built environment, based on the evolving evidence base on effective interventions, would be useful in the future. Examples could include walkability, the proportion of the population close to public transit, the density of green and recreational spaces, etc. The LHIs in this area are limited and are only proxies for a broader range of environmental quality issues.

A review of the literature substantiates the associations between air pollution and poor health outcomes (for example, Henschel et al., 2012). Air Quality Index (AQI) "reports five most common ambient air pollutants that are regulated under the Clean Air Act: ground-level ozone, particle pollution (or particulate matter), carbon monoxide, sulfur dioxide, and nitrogen dioxide" (EPA, 2012[3]). Although the AQI data (collected through the Environmental Protection Agency's monitoring networks) are of high quality, the AQI has considerable geospatial limitations. For example, rural areas are generally not well represented. Also, given the placement of monitors (away from sources of high air pollution), the data collected may not be informative about the cumulative burden of air pollution in a certain area (California Department of Public Health, 2010). The *Guide to Community Preventive Services* has recommended multitrigger and multi-component interventions for asthma control, which would suggest that a composite measure of asthma-aggravating aspects of the environment could be helpful (housing quality in a given area, combined with air quality, and other factors). For air quality, an environmental quality index that can be used for rural and urban areas would be most useful at the local level. At the federal and state level, metrics such as proportion of vehicles that meet a miles-per-gallon threshold could be used.

The logic model provides an illustration of some of the potential areas for measurement related to the AQI indicator. (Children's exposure to secondhand smoke is covered to some extent in the Tobacco Use logic

---

[3] See http://www.epa.gov/o3healthtraining/aqi.html (accessed June 27, 2013).

model earlier in this chapter.) The available literature shows that the AQI is not the only available indicator in this area. The environment is one area where the local, state, and federal needs for quality measures (and the ability to act) may diverge greatly. In other words, the system inputs for environmental quality can be expanded beyond just air quality to also include water, housing, transportation, land use, and food, although data availability and measures may vary widely in each domain. For example, the built environment is an important determinant of health and of great local relevance, but it is harder to identify suitable measures of the built environment. There are several reasons for this. First, although the association between the built environment and health outcomes has support in the literature, the evidence base regarding effective interventions is incomplete and evolving. The *Community Guide* does provide recommendation on several types of interventions on the built environment (e.g., community scale urban design and land use) that are likely to have effects on physical activity.

In the area of indoor air quality, specifically, children's exposure to secondhand smoke (SHS) (the second LHI in this topic), the UK National Institute for Clinical Excellence has found review-level evidence of effectiveness for the several classes of interventions (Taylor et al., 2005). A Cochrane review has also found sufficient evidence of effectiveness for legislative bans on smoking in workplaces and other indoor spaces, with evidence of great effectiveness of bans in hospitals (Callinan et al., 2010). Little evidence is available on policies banning smoking in multi-unit housing, although such policies have been enacted in some jurisdiction on the assumption that they could potentially lower SHS exposure for children.

NQF has endorsed one measure pertinent to secondhand smoke exposure of children inside the home. This is a measure developed by the Maternal and Child Health Bureau of HRSA.

Each community, state, or measure-endorsing entity could use the logic model described below to generate a portfolio of measures for comparison and improvement in the area of environmental quality. The logic model can also be used to assess local resources and capacities to implement interventions to improve air quality.

Air Quality: Example Measures of Quality

The list below provides a partial set of potential measures. Figure 3-4 illustrates how the logic model can be applied to this LHI topic.

Measures of Outcome

Mortality due to respiratory complications
Asthma incidence in children
Inhaler use (as proxy for frequency of asthma attacks)
Hospital visits for asthma attacks
Emergency visits with respiratory related complications

Measures of Healthy Conditions (e.g., Intermediate Outcome)

Concentration of air pollutants in the air
Number of clean air days
Indoor air quality at home and workplace
Mass transit system coverage and use

Measures of Resources (Structure) or Interventions (Process)

Implementation of pollution reduction technology
Proportion of vehicles on the road that meet Corporate Average Fuel
    Economy (CAFE) standards

The following are measures that have been endorsed by NQF (measure steward provided in parentheses). They pertain largely to the clinical care setting and to a far lesser extent to the population level.

- Asthma Emergency Department Visits (Alabama Medicaid Agency)
- Relative Resource Use for People with Asthma (NCQA)

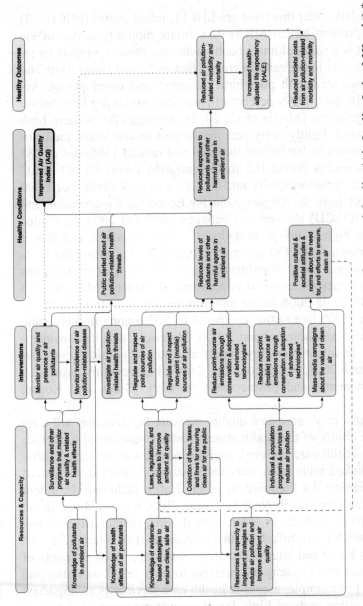

FIGURE 3-4 Applying the logic model to the LHI topic Environmental Quality (Air Quality Index LHI only).*

* Examples of reducing point source emissions include reduces power consumption through conservations measures; replacement of coal and other fossil fuel power generation with water-, wind-, and solar-based power generation; and use of low-sulfur coal, and scrubbers to reduce pollutants in power plant emissions. Examples of reducing mobile sources of air pollution include improvements in fuel efficiency through Corporate Average Fuel Economy standards and reductions in diesel fuel–related emissions through the use of low-sulfur diesel fuel and particulate filters.

Maternal, Infant, and Child Health

The two LHIs under this topic are LHI 11, infant deaths (MICH-1.3) and LHI 12, preterm births (MICH-9.1). Infant mortality is one of the four LHIs that is also an ultimate health outcome. Preterm birth is an intermediate outcome in the causal network that ends with infant death and is strongly associated with poor birth outcomes and development. According to 2010 data, 11.99 percent of American babies are born before 37 weeks of gestation (Martin et al., 2012). Although the preterm birth rate has decreased slightly every year for the past several years, the United States continues to lag behind its peers and ranked 130th out of 184 countries in a recent World Health Organization report (WHO et al., 2012). The U.S. infant mortality rate in 2009 was 6.39 deaths per 1,000 births. A report from the Organisation for Economic Co-operation and Development (OECD) showed that between 2005 and 2009 the United States had the highest infant mortality of 17 peer nations, and that it ranked 31st among 40 OECD countries (OECD, 2011). Within the United States, ethnic and racial disparities in neonatal and infant mortality are deep and persist across levels of educational attainment (Mathews and McDorman, 2012). In 2008, infant mortality among non-Hispanic blacks was 12.67 per 1,000 live births, compared to 5.52 among non-Hispanic whites (Mathews and MacDorman, 2012). Moreover, despite considerable decreases in infant mortality across all socioeconomic groups between 1969 and 2001, socioeconomic deprivation remains associated with higher neonatal and postneonatal mortality (Singh and Kogan, 2007).

Infant deaths may serve as a quality measure because they are a reflection of the ability of the health system (broadly conceived to include public health, health care delivery, social services, and others) to influence factors linked with infant survival at various points in the causal network. Reviewing the literature on infant deaths, including the extensive information provided in *Healthy People 2020*, the committee found that the top causes include, in order: birth defects, prematurity and low birth weight, and Sudden Infant Death Syndrome (SIDS) (Heron, 2012).

Given this broad and interrelated array of causal factors, a variety of system resources and capacity are relevant to both infant mortality and preterm birth. For example, access to health care services is an important factor in preventing preterm birth, but insurance coverage of maternity services is not enough. More than half of women who receive Medicaid coverage of pregnancy and birth lose that coverage within 60 days of giving birth (Johnson, 2012). The loss of coverage has serious consequences for women with medical risks who had previous adverse pregnancy outcomes such as preterm birth or low birth weight, in part because of the likelihood that they will have similar poor outcomes with subsequent births.

A range of social, physical environmental, and economic conditions and changes in behavioral risk factors relate to infant mortality and preterm birth. However, there are considerable gaps in the evidence base. The existing evidence-based interventions to address one or more of the causes of infant mortality and preterm birth include: folic acid supplementation, tobacco use cessation counseling, tobacco use interventions used in combination (excise taxes, campaigns, education) and worksite programs to control and reduce obesity (Community Preventive Services Task Force, 2013). In addition to those lifestyle factors, preterm birth and infant death are also related to teenage and unintended pregnancy, socioeconomic status, educational status of the parents, sleep position, obesity, nutritional status, and infections in the mother, including sexually transmitted diseases (STDs). Clinical interventions that have been effective in addressing causes of infant mortality related to preterm birth include appropriate use of surfactant for preterm neonates experiencing respiratory distress.

A perinatal conceptual risk framework has been proposed, which involves recognizing that although many of the existing interventions occur at the level of the most proximal determinants—risk factors for poor pregnancy outcomes—the foundations for those poor outcomes are laid much earlier in life (Johnson et al., 2006; Misra et al., 2003). Such a life-course framework calls for undertaking strategies at the population and individual levels that intervene much earlier in life, years before a woman conceives, as well as during the interconception periods, with the intent of influencing such factors as nutritional status, tobacco use, and sexual behavior, among many others. Such an array of interventions would require changes in policies, including reorientation of federal and state investments, and the implementation of evidence-based interventions on many fronts. Several recent efforts have sought to improve infant health and survival, including the Association of State and Territorial Health Officials Healthy Babies Initiative, which has carried out efforts to improve birth outcomes in a number of states (ASTHO, 2012); the Peer-to-Peer State Medicaid Learning Project, operated by CDC and the Commonwealth Fund (Johnson, 2012), and the Strong Start for Mothers and Newborns Initiative, which is a joint effort of CMS, HRSA, and the Administration on Children and Families. The Strong Start initiative aims to reduce preterm birth and improve infant and maternal outcomes through two strategies: the reduction of elective deliveries before 39 weeks, and the testing of approaches to reducing prematurity among Medicaid and Children's Health Insurance Program recipients at risk of premature birth.

Maternal, Infant, and Child Health: Example Measures of Quality

The list below provides a partial set of potential measures. Figure 3-5 (page 75) illustrates how the logic model can be applied to this LHI topic.

Measures Related to Healthy Outcomes

Infant mortality rate
Percent of overweight and obesity in pregnant women and women of
    childbearing age
Number of stillbirths and miscarriages
Number of preterm births
Number of children with congenital conditions
Percent of early elective deliveries

Measures Related to Healthy Conditions

Prevalence of infant exposure to environmental tobacco smoke in the
    home (HHS, 2006)
The existence of laws related to indoor air quality, such as municipal
    ordinances prohibiting or restricting smoking in multi-family
    housing (Environmental Law Institute, 2013)
Prevalence of back-to-sleep practices (data from Pregnancy Risk As-
    sessment Monitoring System);
Rate of elective deliveries occurring prior to 39 weeks (objective of
    the National Priorities Partnership)
The rate of overweight and obesity in women of childbearing age
    and in pregnant women
Percentage of women of childbearing age receiving family planning
    services
Percent of pregnant women receiving prenatal care
Number of women that adhere to dietary and nutritional guidelines
    during pregnancy
Percentage of women smoking during pregnancy
Percentage of women who consume alcohol during pregnancy

Percentage of teenage pregnancies

Percentage of unwanted pregnancies

Percentage of women breastfeeding a minimum of 12 months (American Academy of Pediatrics) or 2 years (World Health Organization)

Percentage of infants and children exposed to secondhand smoke

Percentage of vaccinated (up to date) infants and children

Percentage of mothers following nutritional guidelines

Percentage of infants visiting the emergency room

Measures Related to Resources and Interventions

Availability of prenatal care

Availability of family planning services

The following are measures that have been endorsed by NQF (measure stewards provided in parentheses). They pertain largely to the clinical care setting and to a far lesser extent to the population level (e.g., AHRQ).

- Percentage of low-birth-weight births (CDC)
- Low-birth-weight rate (AHRQ)
- Healthy-term newborn (California Maternal Quality Care Collaborative)
- Prenatal and postpartum care (NCQA)
- Infant under 1,500 g not delivered at appropriate level of care (CA Maternal Quality Care Collaborative)
- SIDS counseling
- Exclusive breast milk feeding during the newborn's entire hospitalization (Joint Commission)
- Frequency of ongoing prenatal care (NCQA)
- Prenatal and postpartum care—timeliness of prenatal care and postpartum care at 21 and 56 days after delivery (NCQA)

Given the role of smoking in influencing several factors that lead to infant death, quality measures related to tobacco use may be useful.

- Medical assistance with smoking and tobacco use cessation (three-component—advice to quit, discussion of medications, discussion of strategies for cessation) (NCQA)

- Percentage of patients aged 18 years and older who were screened for tobacco use at least once during the 2-year measurement period *and* who received tobacco cessation counseling intervention if identified as a tobacco user (AMA-convened Physician Consortium for Performance Improvement)
- The HRSA Maternal and Child Health Bureau measures children exposed to secondhand smoke inside their homes (fits under Healthy Conditions).

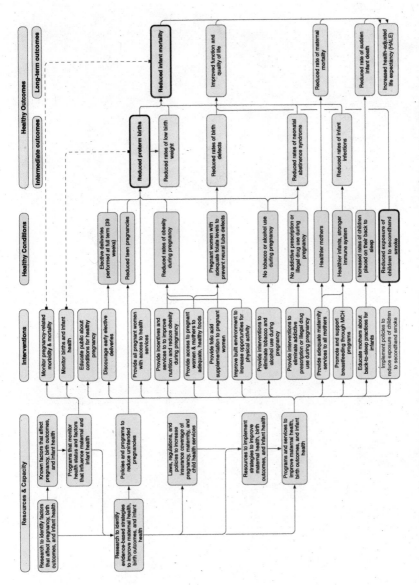

FIGURE 3-5 Applying the logic model to the LHI topic Maternal, Infant, and Child Health.

4

Using the Quality Measures

In this chapter, the committee discusses the use of measures of quality in the context of the implementation of Affordable Care Act (ACA) provisions such as the call for establishing accountable care organizations (ACOs) and changes in community-benefit requirements for nonprofit hospitals; the evolution in public health practice (e.g., a national accreditation movement); the diffusion of the concept of population health within the health care delivery system; and fiscal constraints that motivate the drive to demonstrate quality in terms of value realized on investment. The chapter's primary focus on health care and public health is not intended to suggest that there are no other stakeholders. It is a reflection of the most obvious locus for collaboration to improve the health of communities, and of common ground, such as the fact that many health departments provide clinical care services, and the fact that several provisions of the ACA offer further opportunities for health care delivery and public health practice to "meet in the middle" (see, for example, Stoto [2013]).

When applying the Public Health Quality Forum's definition of quality, particularly the notion of "conditions in which the population can be healthy," to the *Healthy People 2020* Leading Health Indicators (LHIs), it is clear that quality in non-health sectors matters in improving population health. Although the committee was not constituted to examine in detail issues related to measurement in non-health fields, the committee believes that the selection criteria and measures of quality discussed in this report may have broader usefulness, such as to schools, community development financial institutions, and non-health government agencies. Other entities that work in the population health improvement "space" but that may not have health as a primary objective could find measures helpful in documenting co-benefits—for example, areas where improve-

77

ment in health has been associated with improvements in school performance, or where community development and health have strengthened one another. One high-profile example can be found at the intersection of climate change and environmental quality, where policy changes to reduce greenhouse gas emissions can improve air quality, thus improving health outcomes (lower-respiratory and cardiovascular morbidity and mortality) (see, for example, Haines et al., 2009). Another example is the way in which improving the quality of the educational system may be a contributor to increased high school graduation rates (LHI AH-5.1[1]), which, in turn, may have positive health effects. Also, communities where cross-sector coalitions work to improve health (while achieving other socially valuable objectives) may wish to consider a small number of health-oriented measures as a way to measure quality of the collaborative efforts to improve health while strengthening public transit or facilitating healthful community development. A municipality could, for example, report annually on its cross-sector efforts to improve health, using metrics that, like high school graduation rates, go beyond health outcomes and track dimensions of the environment that are known to have health effects.

As outlined in the 2012 Institute of Medicine (IOM) report *For the Public's Health: Investing in a Healthier Future*, the United States obtains low value from its health care delivery system, which is exceptionally high-cost and achieves relatively poor health outcomes compared to other high-income countries. Health care costs have been rising steeply for some time, although a slight slowdown was reported in early 2013 (Cutler and Sahni, 2013; Ryu et al., 2013; Stremikis et al., 2011). Earlier IOM reports have explained how a multisectoral health system can improve population health and increase the value realized on the nation's investment (IOM, 2011a, 2012). The engagement of many sectors is essential to address the well-described multifactorial causes of poor health at the population level (Remington and Booske, 2011). Speakers at the committee's December 2012 information-gathering meeting motivated the committee to focus on the relationship between health care and pub-

---

[1] The complete list of *Healthy People 2020* objectives and approximately 1,200 measures is available from the Healthy People website. Measures are denoted by an acronym for the given *Healthy People 2020* topic (e.g., AH denotes Adolescent Health) and are numbered sequentially according to topic and objective (e.g., AH-5.1, where objective 5 in the topic of Adolescent Health is "increase educational achievement" and measure 5.1 is "Increase the proportion of students who graduate with a regular diploma 4 years after starting 9th grade." The complete list of objectives and measures is available at http://www.healthypeople.gov/2020/topics objectives2020/pdfs/HP2020objectives.pdf (accessed March 4, 2013).

lic health as central among other potential linkages and partnerships for improving population health (see Appendix C). Although recognizing the importance of other stakeholders in the health system, the committee was guided by this central relationship in outlining the uses of quality measures.

There are a growing number of opportunities to use measures of quality. *Healthy People 2020* is directed at the country's entire health enterprise—not merely at governmental public health agencies, but also at health care delivery organizations at all levels, at community-based organizations involved in health improvement, at the business community, at government agencies working in areas relevant to health (e.g., transportation and education) and at many others who contribute in the broadly conceptualized health system described in Chapter 1. The concept of multiple determinants of health was central in the development of *Healthy People 2020* and is reflected in a small way in the 26 LHIs, as some of them are in the purview of health care delivery system, while others (high school graduation rates, depression in adolescents, air quality) are influenced by a wider array of actors, including health departments, schools, community-based organizations, the business sector, and many others.

In describing the uses and users of measures of quality, it is important to clarify some key concepts. The starting point is the concept of "total population" defined by Jacobson and Teutsch (2012) as all persons living within a geopolitical area;[2] this is in contrast to more limited subpopulations, such as the enrollees in a health plan or the patients of a provider. The notion of a system-within-a-system may be useful here, as health care delivery systems, the education system, employer systems, and other systems can be thought of as subsystems, each with its own subpopulation, all of which contribute to total population health. Finally, the distinction between governmental public health infrastructure and the multisectoral health system discussed in Chapter 1 is further illustrated in Figure 4-1. The 2011 IOM report *For the Public's Health: The Role of Measurement in Action and Accountability* updated the work of an earlier IOM committee to create an illustration of government public health as one of many actors contributing to a broader system of assurance for

---

[2] Jacobson and Teutsch (2012) recommend that "the concept and definition of 'total population' and 'total population health' across a specified geopolitical area should be used when setting goals and objectives for improving overall health status and health outcomes of interest to the clinical care system, the government public health system, and stakeholder organizations" (p. 11).

The Public Health System (IOM, 2003a)

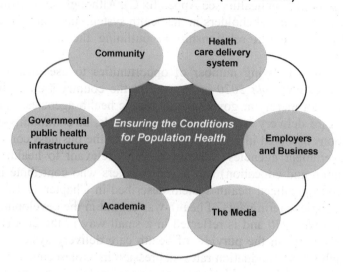

The Health System (IOM, 2011a)

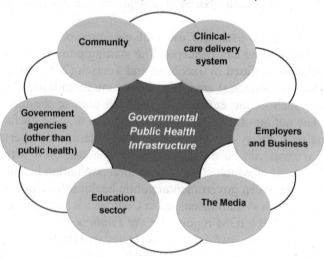

FIGURE 4-1 The multisectoral health system.
SOURCES: IOM, 2003a, 2011a.

population health. The revised illustration, shown in Figure 4-1, places governmental public health infrastructure at the center of the process for population health improvement in acknowledgment of the special responsibility and qualifications of public health agencies in general. However, there are limitations to other stakeholders' ability or willingness to engage, and this illustration reflects an aspiration and not always the reality of the actual functioning of the public health agency as convener, steward of the community's health, knowledge generator and disseminator, and adviser or catalyst in mobilizing to improve health (IOM, 2012).

Viewed through the expansive lens just described, there are many potential users of measures of quality. In addition to governmental public health agencies and communities, health-focused nonprofit and community-based organizations, hospitals and health care systems, ACOs, managed care organizations and payers, and patient-centered medical homes and physician practices all seek the same outcome: to achieve longer, healthier lives for all individuals and populations. The committee hopes that the measure selection criteria and suggested measures of quality in this report will prove to be a useful guide to all who work to improve population health—and especially those who do so in collaboration.

There are numerous recent developments that create opportunities for collaboration that is informed by measures of quality. These developments include the ACA provision that revised the Internal Revenue Service's (IRS's) requirements for tax-exempt hospitals to include conducting a community health needs assessment, the ACA's promotion of accountable care organizations as a governance tool for coordinated and high-quality care, the growing influence of the Three-Part Aim framework, and the creation of a national public health accreditation program that requires state and local public health agencies to conduct health needs assessments and develop improvement plans.

The committee has identified some of the primary users and purposes for the quality measures. Measures can be used (1) by governmental public health agencies; (2) by nonprofit hospitals, ACOs, and other health care entities; (3) by community organizations, philanthropies, and others in their measurement and quality improvement efforts; and (4) for expanding the understanding of the Three-Part Aim. As previously discussed, measures can be used for three purposes:

1. Assessment: providing a snapshot in time, such as community health needs assessments or benchmarking (for the purpose of public reporting, ranking, comparisons, etc.).
2. Improvement: requiring measurement over time, such as assessing progress toward goals in community health improvement efforts.

3. Accountability: demonstrating that investments have been used effectively and efficiently to deliver results (healthy outcomes).

The committee recognizes that these different uses involve somewhat different requirements for data collection and reporting. The present report and chapter focus largely on the use of measures for quality improvement in response to the charge given by the Department of Health and Human Services (HHS).

USE BY GOVERNMENTAL PUBLIC HEALTH AGENCIES

Community health assessments (CHAs) are frequently conducted by public health agencies as part of their community health improvement processes, or in response to state law. CHAs ideally emerge from a community process and are based on knowing which interventions work and how well they work, and they need to be paired with improvement plans in order to address the issues identified. Community health improvement planning is a common activity of local and state health departments, and a quick search of the Web results in hundreds of examples of community health improvement plans developed by an array of jurisdictions and organizations. The National Association for County and City Health Officials (NACCHO) has supported such activities for decades, developing and refining assessment tools such as the Assessment Protocol for Excellence in Public Health (APEX PH) and more recently Mobilizing for Action through Planning and Partnerships (MAPP) (NACCHO, 2007).

Conducting CHAs is a prerequisite for state and local public health agencies to initiate national voluntary accreditation by the Public Health Accreditation Board (PHAB). The development of community and state health improvement plans is another prerequisite for public health accreditation. PHAB was formed to implement and oversee national accreditation of public health departments, with goals that include "to promote high performance and continuous quality improvement" (PHAB, 2011). The first major domain of the accreditation process is assessment, which includes systematic monitoring of health status; the collection, analysis, and dissemination of data; the use of data to inform public health policies, processes, and interventions; and participation in a process for the development of a shared, comprehensive health assessment of the community.

The MAPP tool developed by NACCHO and used by many local health departments includes a four-part process:

1. Community themes and strengths assessment
2. The local public health system assessment
3. The community health status assessment
4. The "forces of change" assessment

A specific application of MAPP is the Community Balanced Scorecard (CBSC) which is a strategic planning process to focus on priority public health outcomes. CBSC can improve the use of MAPP assessments, making MAPP strategies and plans better focused. These processes reinforce the role of governmental public health agencies in leading the assessment of the health of the public for a given community. A robust set of measures of quality provide a solid foundation for these activities.

The Missouri Information for Community Assessment Priority Setting Model (MICA) illustrates one way to prioritize the implementation of a community health improvement plan and "is intended to provide high-level consideration of the diseases or risk factors that are most important to a community" (Simoes et al., 2006). MICA uses data from vital records, hospital discharge records, emergency departments, risk factors from the Behavioral Risk Factor Surveillance System, and eight epidemiologic measures to construct six criteria for setting priorities for community action: size, severity, urgency, preventability, community support, and racial disparity. More recent efforts for planning and prioritization have been undertaken using America's Health Rankings for data at the state level and the County Health Rankings at the county level.

The committee views the nine characteristics of quality in public health identified by the HHS Public Health Quality Forum as a guide for state and community health improvement plans and their implementation. The committee also notes that there is considerable overlap between these nine aims or characteristics and the six improvement aims outlined for health care in the IOM's (2001) *Crossing the Quality Chasm* report. Communicating about this and other areas of convergence could help inform and facilitate joint population health improvement efforts involving health care and public health entities.

Assessment and planning are necessary, but not sufficient for improvement. Furthermore, the complex problems that top the list of priorities identified in most health assessments, such as tobacco use and obesity, cannot be addressed by health departments alone, and, in addition, those agencies do not have sufficient resources to address these issues on their own (IOM, 2012). One promising opportunity for partnership has been created by the revised community benefit obligation of tax-exempt hospitals, which are required to address community needs identified in their newly required community health needs assessments (CHNAs). In the context of existing or new collaborative needs assessment efforts, hospitals can contribute ideas, strategies, and resources (including funding and data).

USE BY NONPROFIT HOSPITALS
AND OTHER HEALTH CARE INSTITUTIONS

According to the IRS, "providing community benefit is required for hospitals to be tax-exempt charitable organizations under section 501(c)(3) of the Internal Revenue Code." Community benefit requirements for tax-exempt hospitals call on institutions to be "transparent, concrete, measurable, and both responsive and accountable to identified community need" (HHS, 2011). Young and colleagues (2013) have shown that hospitals have often used the community benefit requirement to cover uncompensated care, pay for training, and perform other such activities, some of which provide little or very narrowly defined benefits to communities. To accomplish a transformation in the implementation of community benefit requirements, the ACA requires tax-exempt hospitals to conduct a CHNA and to adopt and use an "implementation strategy." Hospitals are required to make the CHNA "widely available to the public" and to report to the IRS on the activities undertaken to respond to the needs identified in the CHNA. Rosenbaum and Margulies (2011), Trust for America's Health (2013), and others have commented on the opportunities afforded by the ACA amendment to the Internal Revenue Code, but they have also called for more specific requirements from the IRS to clarify what is expected of hospitals. One challenge has been the fact that the original regulations ask that hospitals include public health expertise in the assessment, but there was no requirement for hospitals to work with their local public health agency. One potential leverage point is the role of states in cases where the state health agency provides hospitals with certificates of need, in which case the state agency could require that the hospital collaborate with the local public health agency. Nevertheless, this IRS requirement has tremendous potential to facilitate collaboration in the multisectoral health system, and especially between public health and clinical care, to improve population health. Such collaborations can benefit from the framework provided by the Three-Part Aim described later in this chapter.

There are many examples of hospitals contributing to improving population health. Nonprofit hospitals in San Francisco, for example, have been collaborating with the health department for nearly two decades, have been reporting on their community benefit through a shared website since 2007, and have been contributing to the San Francisco Community Health Improvement Plan, due to be completed in 2013. Collaborative efforts have also engaged business and community organizations, and currently the city-wide coalition among hospitals, the public health agency, and other partners is working to "increase healthy living environments, increase healthy eating and physical activity, and increase access to high quality health care and services" (RWJF, 2012). The coalition website provides access to "Community Vital Signs, which makes use of more than 30 data indicators and has set 10 priority health goals that will be measured every year to track their progress" (RWJF, 2012). In another example, Boston Children's Hospital uses nurse practitioners and community health workers to conduct home visits of asthma patients and help identify and remove asthma triggers that are present in the home (Boston Children's Hospital, 2013). The program has resulted in savings in health care costs from decreased emergency room visits, and the hospital has been working with the state Medicaid organization and other payers to develop a payment system for this type of comprehensive preventive approach. Nationwide Children's Hospital in Columbus provides another example of a hospital's community benefits, which it achieves through its "Healthy Neighborhoods, Healthy Families (HNHF), a partnership with the city and community-based organizations to address affordable housing, healthy food access, education, safe and accessible neighborhoods, and workforce and economic development" (Prevention Institute, 2013). The hospital's efforts have contributed seed funding and a partnership with a community development nonprofit organization that led to the addition of more than 100 affordable and revitalized homes to the community (Nationwide Children's Hospital, 2012).

The data resources and overall approach used by nonprofit hospitals to conduct the required CHNA have become more available in a consensus format through www.chna.org (hosted by www.community commons.org), "a free Web-based platform designed to assist nonprofit organizations, state and local health departments, financial institutions, and other organizations seeking to better understand the needs and assets of their communities, and to collaborate to make measurable improvements in community health and well-being" (Community Commons, 2013). These resources, which include advanced mapping and analysis technology, have been developed as a result of broad consensus of hospital, public health, and community organizations. The committee believes that the process for selecting measures of quality described in this report could prove useful to the process of developing CHNA by providing guidance on the most important things to measure everywhere, and the measures will likely add value for improvement efforts emerging from those assessments.

In addition to the new IRS community benefit requirements, the reforms initiated by the ACA include certification of ACOs under Medicare, which can serve as another potential leverage point or vehicle for engaging hospitals and other health care organizations with public health agencies. The Centers for Medicare & Medicaid Services (CMS) defines ACOs as groups of providers that come together to provide well-coordinated and high-quality care to Medicare beneficiaries. CMS has established incentive mechanisms for ACOs, such as the Medicare Shared Savings program that includes 33 required quality measures, 8 of which relate to clinical prevention, and most of which coincide with LHIs (RTI International and Telligen, 2011). There is little consensus about the extent to which ACOs should be truly accountable for total population health, that is, for the health of all individuals residing in a geopolitical area rather than just for chronic disease management for the enrollees in the ACO (Noble and Casalino, 2013). As one example, the Accountable Care Community of Akron, Ohio, described itself as having a community-wide focus (Austen BioInnovation Institute, 2012).

The committee believes that the notion of accountability for improving total population health appeals to more than just health departments. It is congruent with efforts in the health care delivery sector, including more expansive thinking about mechanisms to engage a broader range of stakeholders in population health improvement. Magnan and colleagues (2012) have described accountable health communities as voluntary regional organizations that focus on health in addition to health care, and that engage local stakeholders, including hospitals, health departments, and community organizations in the collection of data, the setting of goals, the facilitation of system reforms, and the demonstration of proper stewardship of financial resources, including investing in the social and environmental determinants of health. Magnan and colleagues (2012) called for the creation of health outcomes trusts, which would build on existing coalitions, and function as the heart of the accountable health community. The trusts would work with state and local health departments to evaluate measures of health and health care—an effort that would be facilitated by having standardized measures of quality from which to draw.

Some community health improvement efforts are driven by a partnership between health care, public health entities, and entities from other sectors, such as academic institutions. Examples can be found across the country, from Sonoma County, California, to Akron, Ohio.[3] Many such collaborations use websites to engage stakeholders and to share information with communities, including community health needs assessments conducted jointly, hospital community benefit plans, health department reports, and other materials.

USE IN EXPANDING AND UNDERSTANDING
THE THREE-PART AIM

As indicated in Chapter 1, the Triple Aim concept developed by the Institute for Healthcare Improvement (IHI) has not only become an important framework in the U.S. health care delivery system, but it also has been adapted for use in CMS and more broadly in HHS as the Three-Part Aim, including as a framework for the National Quality Strategy.

The Three-Part Aim framework—better care/quality, lower costs, and improved population health—provides an ideal platform for health care and public health collaboration since it is familiar to health care audiences and includes an aim to improve population health. IHI continues to work with dozens of new communities using the related Triple Aim approach. This is likely to generate a rich array of information, including, potentially, innovative approaches that can be disseminated widely across health care settings.

The IHI paper "Measuring the Triple Aim" (Stiefel and Nolan, 2012) discusses measurement for all three dimensions of the Triple Aim including population health. However, the population health measurement component emphasizes primarily clinical measures. Although the model of population health and the corresponding analytic framework used in the IHI paper includes an adaptation of the Evans and Stoddart (1990) model of the social determinants of health, the authors acknowledge that necessary and robust measures for some nonclinical factors are not readily available. This observation echoes some of the findings of the National Quality Forum (NQF) Population Health Endorsement Maintenance Steering Committee that attempted to identify and endorse population health measures as part of the larger NQF process and faced considerable limitations and challenges in its work (Jarris and Stange, 2012).

The committee believes that there is an important opportunity for the quality measures discussed in this present report to augment measure-

---

[3] Examples can be found at http://www.healthysonoma.org and http://www.sonomahealth action.org (accessed June 27, 2013).

ments of the population health component of the Three-Part Aim and to expand the use of that framework.

Specific examples of the use of quality measures in initiatives that are implementing the Three-Part Aim need to be studied and the best practices need to be shared. The example of Sonoma County in California shows how a public health agency can assemble a full spectrum of health status, health behavior, and social determinants data to support an initiative in that community. Such examples can serve as important precedent for future Triple Aim or Three-Part Aim projects.

The committee believes that future success in moving the LHIs depends on the extent to which they can be incorporated into Three-Part Aim initiatives and become used by all organizations that use the Three-Part Aim. An essential first step will be to reach out to key measurement experts as well as groups that have worked on population health improvement as part of a Three-Part Aim initiative and to build on the work and learning to date. In this future work, the focus can be to provide reliable and accessible data sources to inform measures of quality.

> **Finding 4-1: The committee finds that the concept of a Three-Part Aim described in the National Quality Strategy could play a growing and important role in the process of establishing population health as an essential area of focus in transforming health care and health in the United States. The committee also finds that additional development is needed by users of the Three-Part Aim to incorporate evidence-based measures representing social and environmental determinants of health, equity, and the concept of total population health.**

The potential of the Three-Part Aim as a transformative concept could be strengthened if government public health agencies are able to perform the role of conveners and facilitators of stakeholders and advisers in ensuring that community health (needs) assessments are conducted from a total population perspective. Health departments do not always have the structure, size, resources, and capabilities required to rise to the challenge, and potential solutions have been discussed elsewhere (including in IOM, 2011a,b, 2012).

RECOMMENDATION 4-1: The committee recommends that the Department of Health and Human Services convene stakeholders to facilitate the use of measures of quality for the multisectoral health system and their integration into all appropriate activities under the Three-Part Aim with a special focus on the social and environmental determinants, equity, and the concept of total population health.

Areas where measures of quality could be integrated in HHS activities include CMS Innovation Center grant programs, Medicare requirements for ACOs, and Centers for Disease Control and Prevention (CDC) programs such as Community Transformation Grants.

KEY REQUIREMENTS FOR USING QUALITY MEASURES FOR IMPROVING POPULATION HEALTH

The committee recognizes that in many ways the use of measures of quality in order to improve population health is still in its infancy. The committee reviewed the NQF *Guidance for Evaluating the Evidence Related to the Focus of Quality Measurement and Importance to Measure and Report* (2011), the "Measuring the Triple Aim" white paper from IHI (Stiefel and Nolan, 2012), and the criteria developed by the Secretary's Advisory Committee on Health Promotion and Disease Prevention Objectives for 2020 (HHS, 2008). The committee also invited several speakers to share lessons learned from state and national population health improvement efforts (see Appendix C). Ultimately, the committee identified a number of criteria for measures used for the purpose of population health improvement. Some measures currently in use do not meet all the criteria, and this report has outlined a vision for better measures for supporting improvement efforts aimed at population health.

Later in this chapter, the committee provides a brief discussion of some key requirements for the measurement enterprise from the perspective of end users in public health, health care, and other settings. Requirements include local relevance of quality measures (which has time and availability components) and equity, as a guiding principle for all measurement and quality improvement efforts. As an example of the importance of local relevance, a community partnership implementing strategies to reduce childhood obesity would seek to measure the impact of those strategies on obesity prevalence as soon as possible. However, timeliness in measuring such improvement in population health is generally not realistic with existing data sources. Closely related to the need for timeliness is the need for quality measures of processes that are directly linked to the interventions being used to improve population health. Such measures provide more timely feedback than is usually possible with outcome measures. They also help teams and coalitions assess the effectiveness of their implementation. A comprehensive list of process measures is beyond the scope of this committee's work; however, it is important to have such a set of measures tied to evidence-based interventions, while recognizing that at a local level other, more specific measures might also be needed. The number of potential measures is enormous and a top-down approach by a national group would likely generate measures that are of limited benefit to actual circumstances at the practice level. A better approach would be to have a system managed by a national entity harvest good process measures, and evaluate and endorse useful measures generated by frontline improvement efforts of demonstrated effectiveness. However, over time, improvement teams and coalitions could develop measures in areas where there are gaps, test and use such measures, and then submit successful measures to an independent body for consideration and endorsement for broad use, as suggested in Recommendation 2-3.

Another important requirement for quality measures to improve population health is to measure equity by examining health disparities and changes in disparities. This is critical for two reasons. First, many groups attempting to improve population health will explicitly try to reduce disparities, widely accepted as an important health objective in the United States. In addition, even when not attempting to reduce disparities directly, they will need to ensure that they are not worsening disparities while working to improve the health of the overall population. In other words, they would use measures of equity as a "balancing measure," to avoid improving some aspects of a system at the expense of others (Randolph et al., 2009). Thus, teams and coalitions using quality measures for improvement will need to stratify key measures for vulnerable subpopulations, and they will need to have data available that allow stratification.

Quality measures used to improve population health must be available at the national, state, and local levels. The committee recognizes that having data available for quality measures at the local level is the biggest challenge and, not surprisingly, is where the greatest gaps lie. Given the obvious centrality of the local community in public health and clinical practice, and given the fact that most improvement efforts will involve implementation at the local level, the committee's search included the guidelines provided in the University of Kansas Community Tool Box for selecting community-level indicators (University of Kansas, 2013). In addition to the characteristics common to any indicators, such as being statistically measurable, logical or scientifically defensible, and reliable, the developers of the tool box added other characteristics: policy relevant, reflective of community values, and attractive to the local media.

USING MEASURES OF QUALITY
BEYOND THE HEALTH SECTOR

The committee has provided examples of the potential use of measures of quality by health care and public health organizations, but applications of quality measures could extend to philanthropic organizations, business, and non-health government organizations. The processes required for identifying and using measures of quality for assessment, improvement, and accountability may be convened by an "integrator," which is "an entity that serves a convening role and works intentionally and systemically across various sectors to achieve improvements in health and well-being for an entire population in a specific geographic area. Examples of integrators range from integrated health systems and quasi-governmental agencies to community-based non-profits and coalitions" (Chang, 2012). The engagement of non-health stakeholders in efforts to improve health (along with achieving other, primary objectives) has expanded greatly in recent years. Examples from the public sector include the ACA-established National Prevention, Health Promotion, and Public Health Council, which brings together multiple cabinet secretaries and agency heads under the leadership of the Surgeon General, and "health-in-all-policies" efforts such as the joint Sustainable Communities Initiative of the Department Housing and Urban Development, the Department of Transportation, and the Environmental Protection Agency.

A strong knowledge base makes it possible to document the complex and multiple relationships between socioeconomic determinants and health outcomes, and between factors in the built environment and health. Understanding these relationships, and increasingly, some of the interventions that can influence them, requires common ways to measure and report progress. This provides further rationale for community health assessment (and the use of measures of quality as part of such assessments). Various aspects of the built environment—including housing, the accessibility of food and other essential items, opportunities for community entrepreneurs, and the availability of green spaces—are important factors that influence health outcomes, but actions on these factors take place outside the public health and health care sectors. The Community Reinvestment Act (CRA), which is intended to encourage banking institutions to help meet the credit needs of the communities in which they operate, including low- and moderate-income neighborhoods, offers additional uses for community health needs assessments. The CRA regulation contains an option for banks and community development financial institutions to develop a plan with community input detailing how the institution proposes to meet its CRA obligation. The plan is tailored to the needs of the community using direct community input at the development stage, where health care and health concerns can be a major focus. The committee believes that financial institutions can use measures of quality to focus on improving total population health as one of their objectives in community development. The Federal Reserve has been engaged in development efforts, including enhancing the food environment, improving neighborhoods by bringing in small businesses, and strengthening public transit to increase access to employment and other necessities, with a secondary benefit of increased physical activity (as evidence indicates that public transit is linked with more walking) (Erickson and Andrews, 2011).

Investing in What Works for America's Communities: Essays on People, Place & Purpose showcases and discusses the innovations that can be harnessed to transform struggling communities (Andrews and Erickson, 2012, p. 378). The authors describe an approach to community development that is

> focused on leadership that is able to promote a compelling vision of success for an entire community, marshal the necessary resources, and lead people in an integrated way. It must be accountable for outcomes, not just specific outputs (such as the number of apartments built). The outcome goals for the entire community should be bold: doubling the high school graduation rate, halving the number of people living below the poverty line, cutting emergency room visits by 75 percent, or making sure 100 percent of kindergarteners arrive at school ready to learn.

In another example, the Community Development Department of the Federal Reserve Bank of San Francisco conducts a Community Indicators Project "to collect input from community development professionals about the issues and trends facing low- and moderate-income (LMI) communities in the 12th District" (Federal Reserve Bank of San Francisco, 2013). Health was identified as the ninth out of nine top issues, but some of the other issues are linked with the social determinants of health, including household financial stability, the housing market, and employment conditions. It is unclear whether this Federal Reserve project is being used as part of a broader effort to measure and document improvement, but it provides a possible locus for the use of measures of quality to assess the effects of community development efforts on population health improvement.

CONCLUDING OBSERVATIONS

The United States currently receives poor value from its health system, whose investments are largely in the clinical realm. Unsustainably high cost and mediocre outcomes constitute a dual challenge that is having a growing effect on U.S. health and wealth (Johnson, 2012; NRC and IOM, 2013; World Economic Forum, 2008). Substantial progress in improving population health is needed, and quality measures can help public health departments, health care organizations, communities, and many others to work collaboratively to maximize strengths and begin to alter the conditions for health.

It will also be important for HHS and other stakeholders to promote the use of a unified portfolio of measures with the characteristics described in Recommendation 2-1, and that would emerge from the endorsement process across the country and in a range of settings including the clinic and the community. There are specific challenges that need to be addressed first, most notably making timely data available at the local level and identifying better process measures for local use. Addressing these needs as well as taking advantage of the numerous extant and emerging opportunities for multisectoral engagement to improve population health will be vital to the nation's health and well-being for many decades to come.

A

Glossary

Accountable Care Organizations (ACOs): The Centers for Medicare & Medicaid Services defines ACOs as groups of doctors, hospitals, and other health care providers, who come together voluntarily to give co-ordinated high-quality care to their Medicare patients. ACOs have come to hold an even broader meaning, referring to coordinating activities for health care and health for patients of all kinds (e.g., not just Medicare) and for communities in general, as described by the related concepts of Accountable Care Communities and Accountable Health Communities (Austen BioInnovation Institute, 2012; Magnan et al., 2012).

Healthy conditions: The committee used this term in reference to the Department of Health and Human Services (HHS) definition of quality in public health reference to "conditions in which people can be healthy," denoting the determinants of health or factors influencing health. These also correspond to intermediate outcomes.

Healthy People 2020: An effort of HHS, Healthy People "provides science-based, 10-year national objectives for improving the health of all Americans. For 3 decades, Healthy People has established benchmarks and monitored progress over time in order to: encourage collaborations across communities and sectors, empower individuals toward making informed health decisions, and measure the impact of prevention activities."[1]

Leading Health Indicators (LHIs): Twenty-six metrics organized by 12 topics that represent a key set in *Healthy People 2020*, drawn from the more than 1,200 *Healthy People 2020* objectives.

---

[1] See http://www.healthypeople.gov/2020/about/default.aspx (accessed June 13, 2013).

Multisectoral health system: Refers to the array of sectors and entities that influence the health of the population through their activities, ideally in a coordinated manner, as a system, but in practice, operating through occasional and not always sustained collaboration. The system comprises public health agencies, health care delivery organizations, and parts of other sectors (e.g., businesses, schools) and the community (IOM, 2011a). After introducing the term, the report often shortens it to "health system."

National Priorities Partnership: At the behest of HHS, the National Quality Forum (NQF) convened more than 50 public and private organizations in the National Priorities Partnership, which provides annual input to HHS on the implementation of the National Quality Strategy.

National Quality Forum (NQF): The Forum is a nonprofit membership organization that "operates under a three-part mission to improve the quality of American health care by

- building consensus on national priorities and goals for performance improvement and working in partnership to achieve them;
- endorsing national consensus standards for measuring and publicly reporting on performance; and
- promoting the attainment of national goals through education and outreach programs."[2]

National Quality Strategy: In 2010, the Affordable Care Act charged HHS with developing a national quality strategy to "improve the delivery of health care services, patient health outcomes, and population health. After engaging both public and private stakeholders and collecting input, the National Quality Strategy was released in March 2011."[3]

The **nine aims** or the **nine characteristics:** see **Quality characteristics**

Population health: The health of the public in a geopolitical location; see also **Total population health**

---

[2] See http://www.qualityforum.org/About_NQF/About_NQF.aspx (accessed June 27, 2013).
[3] Healthcare.gov factsheet: http://www.healthcare.gov/news/factsheets/2012/04/national-quality-strategy04302012a.html (accessed June 27, 2013).

Public health: In the report, this term refers to governmental public health agencies, also known as health departments, and to their work (public health practice and public health activities).

Public health quality: "The degree to which policies, programs, services, and research for the population increase desired health outcomes and conditions in which the population can be healthy" (Public Health Quality Forum, 2008).

Quality characteristics: Shorthand for the nine aims for improvement of quality in public health *or* characteristics to guide public health practices (Public Health Quality Forum, 2008).

Six drivers: The six priorities for quality improvement in public health (Honoré and Scott, 2010).

Three-Part Aim: The Three-Part Aim is the HHS adaptation of the Institute for Healthcare Improvement's "Triple Aim," and is a conceptual triad of (1) better care, (2) lower cost, and (3) healthy people/healthy communities; see also **Triple Aim**

Total population health: A term developed to distinguish the public health profession's understanding of population health from the narrower interpretation of population health used in the health care delivery sector. Total population health refers to the population in a geopolitical area, while the term "subpopulations" can be used to describe the populations of patients or insured individuals to which practitioners in health care delivery refer.

Triple Aim: Improving the patient experience of care (including quality and satisfaction), improving the health of populations, and reducing the per capita cost of care.[4]

---

[4] See http://www.ihi.org/offerings/Initiatives/TripleAim/Pages/default.aspx (accessed June 13, 2013).

B

Sample Criteria Consulted

TABLE B-1 Previously Published Criteria for Selected Groups of Measures

Category for Criteria	NQF, 2012: Measure evaluation criteria: Criteria for evaluation once measure meets criteria for consideration (NQF, 2012b)	HHS SAC, 2011: Operation criteria for selection of LHIs (HHS, 2008, 2013)	IOM, 2010: Future directions for the national quality Criteria for selecting measures (IOM, 2010)	IOM, 2003b: Priority areas for National Action Criteria for identifying priority areas for health care quality efforts (IOM, 2003)
Criteria that apply to the condition(s) or outcome(s) to be measured				
Impact (Importance)	• Impact: Priority (measure addresses identified priority or has high impact on patients)	• Central: important as a determinant of health status • Instinctive: easily recognized as intimate to health status • Immutable: convey a sense of the obligation to act	• Importance: high-impact based on potential population impact, high cost, variation in quality, low performance levels, or existing disparities • Applicability to national priorities: Does it measure progress in at least one of the national priority areas for improving the quality of health care and eliminating disparities?	• Impact: the extent of the burden—disability, mortality, and economic costs—imposed by a condition, including effects on patients, families, communities, and societies. • Inclusiveness: the relevance of an area to a broad range of individuals with regard to age, gender, socioeconomic status, and ethnicity/race (equity) ... and the breadth of change effected through such strategies across a range of health care settings and providers (reach).

Improvability			
• Impact: opportunity for improvement (i.e., performance gap) • Impact: evidence (measure focus is health outcome or is evidence-based) • Usability and use: extent to which potential audiences are using or could use performance results for both accountability and performance improvement	• Actionable: convey a sense of the possibility to act	• Improvability: is there evidence (not limited to RCTs) that improvement can be made? • Value: does the measure have the potential to increase health care value by narrowing a defined quality gap? • If criteria are met, select measure for use based on its ranking to improve population health and equity	• Improvability: the extent of the gap between current practice and evidence-based best practice and the likelihood that the gap can be closed and condition improved through change in an area; and the opportunity to achieve dramatic improvement in the six national quality aims identified in the Quality Chasm report (safety, effectiveness, patient-centeredness, timeliness, efficiency, and equity). • Inclusiveness: the generalizability of associated quality improvement strategies to many types of conditions and illnesses across the spectrum of health care (representativeness); and the breadth of such strategies across a range of health care settings and providers (reach).

TABLE B-1 Continued

Category for Criteria	NQF, 2012: Measure evaluation criteria: Criteria for evaluation once measure meets criteria for consideration (NQF, 2012b)	HHS SAC, 2011: Operation criteria for selection of LHIs (HHS, 2008, 2013)	IOM, 2010: Future directions for the national quality Criteria for selecting measures (IOM, 2010)	IOM, 2003b: Priority areas for National Action Criteria for identifying priority areas for health care quality efforts (IOM, 2003)
Criteria that apply to the condition(s) or outcome(s) to be measured				
Scientific soundness	• Validity • Reliability: measure is well defined and precisely specified and produces same results when repeated • Comparison to related measures to ensure harmonization		• Sound measure available: Have scientifically sound measures been developed to assess this area?	
Geographic, temporal, and population coverage		• Divisible: into key sub-populations • Translatable: to the national, state, community, and individual levels • Measurable: at a point in time, over time	• Equity: does the measure document significant inequities in care by race, ethnicity, language need, or socioeconomic status? • Geographic and health systems equity: does the measure document	• Inclusiveness: the relevance of an area to a broad range of individuals with regard to age, gender, socio-economic status, and ethnicity/race (equity) … and the breadth of change effected through such strategies across a range of health care settings and providers (reach).

103

Data availability

geographic or health system variation in performance?

- Feasibility: data are readily available or could be captured without undue burden and can be implemented for performance measurement

- Data availability: Does an appropriate national data source exist that would support assessment of performance overall as well as among disparity populations?

C

Meeting Agenda

**Meeting of the IOM Committee on Quality Measures
for the Healthy People Leading Health Indicators**

December 10, 2012

AGENDA

Location:
NAS Building
2101 Constitution Avenue, NW
Washington, DC
Room 120

10:00 a.m.   Welcome and introductions

Steven Teutsch
IOM Committee Chair

10:15 a.m.   Giving of the charge

Howard Koh
Assistant Secretary for Health
Department of Health and Human Services (HHS)

Peggy Honoré
Director, Public Health System, Finance, and
*   Quality Program*
Office of the Assistant Secretary for Health
HHS

10:55 a.m.   Questions from the committee

11:25 a.m.   A perspective on quality measurement in health care

> *Mary Barton*
> *Vice President, Performance Management*
> *National Committee for Quality Assurance*

11:45 a.m.   Questions from the committee

12:00 p.m.   Lunch

1:00 p.m.   Quality measurement at the interface of health care and population health

> *Shari Ling*
> *Deputy Chief Medical Officer*
> *Office of Clinical Standards and Quality*
> *Centers for Medicare & Medicaid Services*

> *John Auerbach*
> *Professor of Practice*
> *Director, Institute of Urban Health Research*
> *Northeastern University*
> *Former Massachusetts Commissioner of Public*
>   *Health and Co-Chair, Massachusetts Statewide*
>   *Quality Advisory Committee*

> *Sanne Magnan*
> *Executive Director*
> *Institute for Clinical Systems Improvement*

2:00 p.m.   Questions from the committee

2:25 p.m.   Break

2:35 p.m.   Developing public health quality indicators: From practical approaches to specific topics

> *Greg Randolph*
> *Director, NC Center for Public Health Quality*
> *Associate Professor of Pediatrics*
> *University of North Carolina*

Rohit Ramaswamy
Director, Center for Global Learning
Clinical Associate Professor
Public Health Leadership Program
University of North Carolina

Abraham Wandersman
Professor, Department of Psychology
University of South Carolina

3:35 p.m.   Questions from the committee

An update from the National Quality Forum Population
Health: Prevention Endorsement Maintenance Steering
Committee

Paul Jarris
Executive Director
Association of State and Territorial Health Officials
Co-Chair of the Steering Committee

Kurt Stange
Professor of Family Medicine, Epidemiology &
*   Biostatistics, Sociology, and Oncology*
Case Western Reserve University
Co-Chair of the Steering Committee

4:40 p.m.   Questions from the committee

5:00 p.m.   Adjourn

D

Committee Biosketches

Steven M. Teutsch, M.D., M.P.H. (*Chair*), became the Chief Science Officer, Los Angeles County Department of Public Health, in February 2009 where he will continue his work on evidence-based public health and policy. He had been in Outcomes Research and Management program at Merck since October 1997 where he was responsible for scientific leadership in developing evidence-based clinical management programs, conducting outcomes research studies, and improving outcomes measurement to enhance quality of care. Prior to joining Merck he was Director of the Division of Prevention Research and Analytic Methods (DPRAM) at Centers for Disease Control and Prevention (CDC) where he was responsible for assessing the effectiveness, safety, and the cost-effectiveness of disease and injury prevention strategies. DPRAM developed comparable methodology for studies of the effectiveness and economic impact of prevention programs, provided training in these methods, developed CDC's capacity for conducting necessary studies, and provided technical assistance for conducting economic and decision analysis. The Division also evaluated the impact of interventions in urban areas, developed the *Guide to Community Preventive Services*, and provided support for CDC's analytic methods. He has served as a member of that Task Force and the U.S. Preventive Services Task Force, which develops the *Guide to Clinical Preventive Services*, as well as on America's Health Information Community Personalized Health Care Workgroup. He chaired the Secretary's Advisory Committee on Genetics Health and Society, and served on the Evaluation of Genomic Applications in Prevention and Practice Workgroup as well as Institute of Medicine panels. Dr. Teutsch started at CDC in 1977, where he was assigned to the Parasitic Diseases Division and worked extensively on toxoplasmosis. He was then assigned to the Kidney Donor and subsequently the Kidney Disease Program. He developed the framework for CDC's diabetes control program. He joined the Epidemiology Program Office and became the Director of the Division of Surveillance and Epidemiology where he was responsible for CDC's disease monitoring activities. He became Chief of the Prevention Effectiveness Activity in 1992. Dr. Teutsch has published more than 150 articles and 6 books in a broad range of fields in epidemiology, including parasitic diseases, diabetes, technology assessment, health services research, and surveillance.

Kevin Grumbach, M.D., is Professor and Chair of the Department of Family and Community Medicine at the University of California, San Francisco (UCSF). He is Co-Director of the UCSF Center for Excellence in Primary Care and Co-Director of the Community Engagement and Health Policy Program for the UCSF Clinical and Translational Science Institute. His research on topics such as primary care physician supply and access to care, innovations in the delivery of primary care, and racial and ethnic diversity in the health professions have been published in major medical journals such as the *New England Journal of Medicine* and *JAMA* and cited widely in both health policy forums and the general media. With Tom Bodenheimer, he co-authored the best-selling textbook on health policy *Understanding Health Policy—A Clinical Approach*, and the book *Improving Primary Care—Strategies and Tools for a Better Practice*, published by McGraw-Hill. He received a Generalist Physician Faculty Scholar award from the Robert Wood Johnson Foundation, the Health Resources and Services Administration Award for Health Workforce Research on Diversity, and the Richard E. Cone Award for Excellence and Leadership in Cultivating Community Partnerships in Higher Education, and is a member of the Institute of Medicine, National Academy of Sciences.

Romana Hasnain-Wynia, Ph.D., is Director, Addressing Disparities, at the Patient-Centered Outcomes Research Institute (PCORI). Dr. Hasnain-Wynia joined PCORI from Northwestern University, where she directed the Center for Healthcare Equity and was Associate Professor at the Feinberg School of Medicine. Prior to her work at Northwestern, Dr. Hasnain-Wynia served as vice president of research for the Health Research and Educational Trust, the research and education affiliate of the American Hospital Association. Dr. Hasnain-Wynia has served as the principal investigator for a number of national studies examining quality of care for underserved populations. She also is a Senior Associate Editor at the journal *Health Services Research*. She received her Ph.D. in health policy from Brandeis University's Heller School for Social Policy and Management.

Jewel Mullen, M.D., M.P.H., M.P.A. In December 2010, Governor Dannel P. Malloy announced his appointment of Dr. Mullen as Commissioner of the Connecticut Department of Public Health (DPH). As Commissioner, Dr. Mullen oversees the state's leading public health agency whose mission is to protect and improve the health and safety of Connecticut residents. Prior to joining the Department, Dr. Mullen was Director of the Bureau of Community Health and Prevention at the Massachusetts DPH. She also is the former medical director of Baystate Mason Square Neighborhood Health Center in Springfield, Massachusetts. Dr. Mullen began her clinical career as a member of the National Health Service Corps at Bellevue Hospital in New York, after which she joined the medical faculty of the University of Virginia. A Connecticut resident since 1992, she has been a member of the medical staff at the Hospital of St. Raphael, the Yale University Health Services, and Yale New Haven Hospital. Board certified in internal medicine, Dr. Mullen received her bachelor and master of public health degrees from Yale University, where she also completed a postdoctoral fellowship in psychosocial epidemiology. A graduate of the Mount Sinai School of Medicine, she completed her residency at the Hospital of the University of Pennsylvania. She also holds a master in public administration degree from the Harvard University John F. Kennedy School of Government. She brings to her role as Commissioner the recognition that efforts to improve the health of individuals and communities must be informed by an understanding of the social context which determines their behaviors and their access to resources.

John Oswald, Ph.D., M.P.H., is Adjunct Assistant Professor in the School of Public Health at the University of Minnesota. While maintaining his academic appointment, he has worked in Washington, DC, over the past 3 years as Assistant Vice President at the National Association of Public Hospitals and Health Systems in 2011 to early 2013 and as Senior Policy Analyst at the Office of Policy at the Centers for Medicare and Medicaid Services in 2010-2011. During this time, he has also been a Lecturer at the Jefferson School of Population Health. Prior to moving to Washington, DC, he was Senior Director of Product Analytics at OptumHealth, a subsidiary of United Healthcare in 2007-2010. Prior to joining OptumHealth, he was the Director of the Center for Health Statistics at the Minnesota Department of Health, where he was responsible from 1993 through 2007 for program evaluation, vital statistics, and health surveys. He was previously from 1983 to 1992 at HealthPartners, a large Minnesota-based health plan in strategic planning and medical management positions. He obtained a Ph.D. in Health Services Research at the University of Minnesota in 1999 and a Master's of Public Health from the University of Minnesota in 1984.

R. Gibson Parrish, M.D., M.P.H., is currently an independent consultant for the Public Health Informatics Institute. Previously, he was Adjunct Associate Professor of Community and Family Medicine at Dartmouth Medical School and Senior Public Health Scientist at the Centers for Disease Control and Prevention (CDC). He is co-author with Daniel Friedman of *Shaping a Health Statistics Vision for the 21st Century*, a report of the National Committee on Vital and Health Statistics, and wrote the recently published article, Measuring Population Health Outcomes. While at CDC, he served in the Epidemiology Program Office and was responsible for overseeing notifiable disease surveillance. He also served in the National Center for Environmental Health, where with Dr. Roy Ing he created the medical examiner surveillance system. Two of the many CDC committees on which Dr. Parrish served were the Surveillance Coordinating Group and the Health Information and Surveillance System Board. He recently served as a member of the Institute of Medicine Committee on Leading Health Indicators for Healthy People 2020.

Greg Randolph, M.D., M.P.H., is Director of the Center for Public Health Quality and is a Professor of Pediatrics and Adjunct Professor of Public Health at the University of North Carolina (UNC) at Chapel Hill. Dr. Randolph has more than 15 years of experience in quality improvement (QI) leadership, implementation, and research. He is currently involved in a range of QI programs and projects, including leading a Centers for Disease Control and Prevention (CDC)-funded project to create a statewide quality improvement infrastructure for the NC public health system, leading a national initiative to develop a Web-based resource to assist public health professionals with implementation of evidence-based interventions, assisting the NC Area Health Education Centers' Statewide Quality Program, and serving as a QI consultant for the American Academy of Pediatrics' Community Pediatrics Training Initiative. He currently provides QI expertise nationally via serving on the Public Health Accreditation Board's Evaluation and Quality Improvement Committee, the American Board of Pediatrics Maintenance of

Certification Committee, the American Academy of Pediatrics (AAP) Steering Committee for Quality Improvement and Management, and as Editor of the *AAP Quality Connections* newsletter. He has published extensively on the application of QI and patient safety in health care and public health. Most recently he served as Guest Editor for the Jan/Feb 2012 *Journal of Public Health Management and Practice* devoted to QI in public health. He has also served as QI faculty for the National Initiative for Children's Healthcare Quality, the New York City Department of Health, and the Institute for Healthcare Improvement. He has assisted the RAND Corporation, University of California, Los Angeles (UCLA), and Cincinnati Children's Hospital with various QI initiatives. Dr. Randolph received his M.D./M.P.H. degree from UNC at Chapel Hill, completed a General Academic Pediatric Fellowship and Preventive Medicine Residency at UNC at Chapel Hill, and is a CDC National Public Health Leadership Institute Scholar.

Patrick Remington, M.D., M.P.H., is Professor of Population Health Sciences and Associate Dean for Public Health at the School of Medicine and Public Health, University of Wisconsin (UW)–Madison. He is nationally recognized for his work in applying epidemiology at the interface between science and practice—culminating in the County Health Rankings, a national program to engage communities in broad-based efforts to mobilize citizens toward actions that improve their health. He graduated Phi Beta Kappa from UW with a degree in molecular biology (1976) and was an Alpha Omega Alpha graduate from the UW Medical School (1981). From 1982 to 1988, he served in the U.S. Public Health Service at the Centers for Disease Control and Prevention (CDC), where he was an Epidemic Intelligence Service Officer, completed a Preventive Medicine Residency, and received his M.P.H. (University of Minnesota) as part of CDC's career development program. While at the CDC, he helped establish the Behavioral Risk Factor Surveillance System now used in every state in the United States. From 1988 to 1997, he was the Chief Medical Officer for Chronic Disease and Injury Prevention in the Wisconsin Division of Health, where he developed and promoted evidence-based interventions in tobacco and breast cancer control, supported by grants from the CDC and the National Cancer Institute. In July 1997, he joined the Department of Population Health Sciences at UW, where his research has focused on methods used to measure the health of communities and communicate this information to the public and policy makers. He is currently co-directing the Robert Wood Johnson Foundation–supported County Health Rankings, a project that ranks the health of the counties in all 50 states and examines strategies to improve population health. He has authored or co-authored more than 220 publications, including the American Public Health Association textbook *Chronic Disease Epidemiology and Control*. As a leader at UW, Dr. Remington established the Population Health Institute, the Master of Public Health Program, and the Comprehensive Cancer Center's Population Health Sciences Program. In 2009, he was appointed the inaugural Associate Dean for Public Health, and is leading an effort to establish the nation's first "transformed school of medicine and public health" integrating public health throughout the school's research, teaching, and service missions. He has received numerous honors recognizing his work, including his selection as the 2010 Langmuir Lecturer at CDC and his appointment to the HHS *Healthy People 2020* Federal Advisory Committee.

Jane E. Sisk, Ph.D., M.A., is a Scholar in Residence at the Institute of Medicine (IOM), Board of Health Care Services. Before the IOM, she served as Director, Division of Health Care Statistics, National Center for Health Statistics, the federal health statistical agency that is part of the Centers for Disease Control and Prevention, from 2004 to 2011. That Division surveys physicians, hospitals, and other health care providers on their organizational arrangements, patients, and clinical care. Since coming to the IOM, Dr. Sisk along with colleagues has drawn from those surveys to publish analyses of physicians' adoption of electronic health records during the past decade, and are analyzing recent changes in physicians' organizational and payment arrangements. She also served on the IOM Committee on Geographic Adjustment in Medicare Payment. Dr. Sisk's research has focused on interventions to improve the quality of care, especially to reduce disparities among population subgroups; evaluation of Medicaid managed care; and the cost-effectiveness of health care interventions, including pneumococcal and influenza vaccinations for elderly people. She was a tenured professor at Mount Sinai School of Medicine, Department of Health Policy, from 1999 to 2009, and at Columbia University, Mailman School of Public Health, Division of Health Policy and Management, Mailman School of Public Health, Columbia University, from 1992 to 1999. Before that, Dr. Sisk was a Senior Associate and Project Director at the Congressional Office of Technology Assessment. She has served on 10 committees at the IOM, from vaccine development to telehealth, and is on three editorial boards. Dr. Sisk holds a Ph.D. in economics from McGill University, and a B.A. in international relations from Brown University. She has been elected a member of the

IOM, National Academy of Sciences; a Fellow of AcademyHealth; and a Fellow of the New York Academy of Medicine.

Pierre Vigilance, M.D., M.P.H., is the Associate Dean for Public Health Practice at the George Washington University School of Public Health and Health Services, where he teaches and advises students, oversees the Practicum program, and provides connectivity with local and regional public health practice activities. He serves on a number of committees, and is routinely engaged in business and strategic partnership development both locally and in the Caribbean. Formerly the Director of the District of Columbia Department of Health, when a new mayoral administration took office in January 2011, Dr. Vigilance departed government service after almost a decade of local public health practice. During his time as the leader of the public health agency for the nation's capital, he led the agency's promotion of health and wellness through innovative physical activity and nutrition projects such as community-level Ward Walks, the Healthy Corner Store Initiative, and Live Well DC. He also supported the development of an ongoing HIV testing, education, and prevention strategy including the Rubber Revolution. Under his leadership, the Department streamlined business processes, adopted a data-driven decision model, and integrated outcome-driven performance management into all practices and initiatives. His focus on telling the story led to the publication of the District's first HIV/AIDS *Epidemiology Reports*; the *Preventable Causes of Death Report* (the first city-level report ever produced); the *Obesity Report*; and the *Obesity Action Plan*. Prior to his appointment in the District of Columbia, Dr. Vigilance served in public health leadership roles in Baltimore City and Baltimore County, Maryland. As Baltimore City's Assistant Health Commissioner, he directed an aggressive HIV outreach and education campaign "Live, Love, Be Safe," which resulted in increased awareness of HIV/AIDS in Baltimore City. He continues to serve as an advocate for expanded access to HIV testing, and de-stigmatization of HIV/AIDS, and participated in the 2010 International AIDS Society conference in Vienna, Austria. Trained in emergency response, his emergency preparedness policy and investigation experience includes Sudden Acute Respiratory Syndrome, tuberculosis, H1N1, multiple vaccination clinics, and local/state preparedness exercises, as well as the public health planning for the 44th Presidential Inauguration. Before entering the government, his work focused on the development of a community-based substance abuse program along with other social justice–oriented community-based interventions in East Baltimore. Dr. Vigilance received his M.D. and M.P.H.

degrees from Johns Hopkins University and is residency-trained in emergency medicine. In addition to George Washington, he has served on faculty at the Johns Hopkins and Georgetown Universities. He is an active member of Alpha Phi Alpha Fraternity, Incorporated, an inductee of the Alpha chapter of Delta Omega at Johns Hopkins University, and a member of Leadership Greater Washington.